THE INSULIN RESISTANCE DIET FOR PCOS

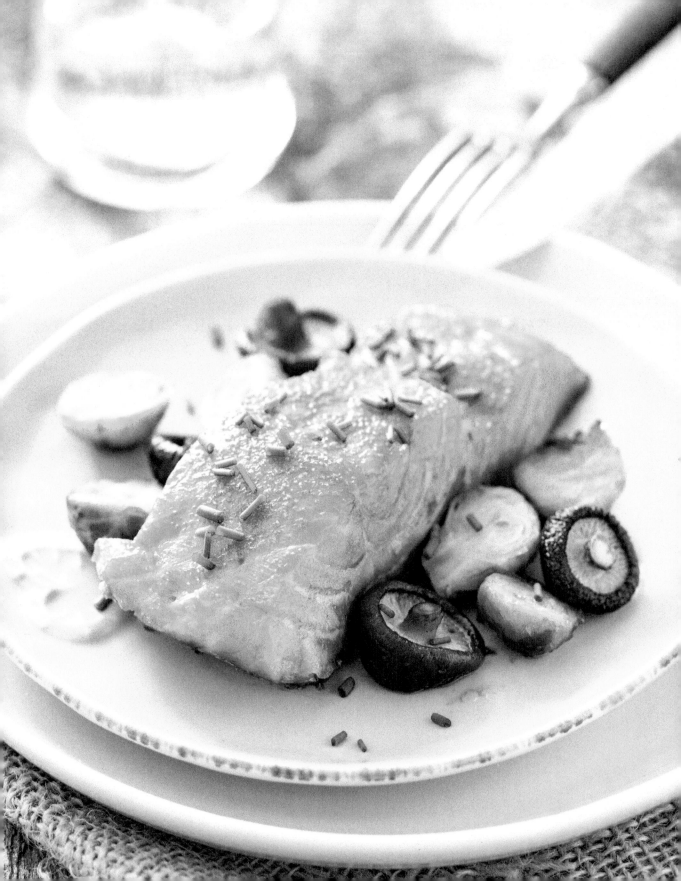

The Insulin Resistance Diet for **PCOS**

A 4-Week Meal Plan and Cookbook to Lose Weight, Boost Fertility, and Fight Inflammation

Tara Spencer and Jennifer Koslo, PHD, RDN

ROCKRIDGE
PRESS

This book is dedicated to the scared women who feel alone; I promise you, you are not.
—Tara

This book is dedicated to my parents, Erma and Walt, who have always been there for me.
—Jennifer

Contents

Introduction

Tara's Story

I had long felt that something was wrong with my body before I was formally diagnosed with polycystic ovarian syndrome (PCOS) and insulin resistance in my early twenties. I only experienced three or four menstrual cycles per year, I could not conquer my painful, cystic acne no matter what medication I took or skin-care products I used, and I seemed to gain weight anytime I even looked at a carbohydrate.

After a couple of years of suffering severe cramps in my abdominal region—which did not seem to be linked to either my diet or my mostly absent menstrual cycle—I finally visited a doctor for blood tests and an ultrasound, to confirm what I already suspected.

At the time of my PCOS diagnosis four years ago, I was preparing for my first bodybuilding competition. Upon researching the condition further, I learned that dropping my body fat levels was the worst thing I could do if I ever hoped to be healthy and fertile, as it would only wreak further hormonal havoc on my body.

I was devastated by the diagnosis. I had been preparing to compete for years, following a strict diet and an all-consuming training regime. Not only did I feel that my personal dreams had been shattered, but I also felt like a fraud working as a personal trainer, since I knew I would never have the expected lean body. Knowing that I could no longer compete made me lose all sense of direction.

Luckily, over time, I used my knowledge as a certified nutritionist to learn how to manage my symptoms naturally, and I found other passions within the fitness industry. I modified my diet, training regime, and general lifestyle, and now I suffer with only the mildest of PCOS symptoms. Most positively, I have completely overcome my insulin resistance, which I credit for the marked improvement in my other symptoms.

In a way, my PCOS diagnosis was a blessing in disguise, because I have discovered numerous things about my body I never would have known otherwise. I am more in tune with my body and now realize the important roles diet and stress management play in ensuring optimal health. I also have greater appreciation of the connection between having a positive body image, practicing self-compassion, and managing a medical condition.

My own personal experiences led me to coach other women who experience the same feelings of confusion, fear, and disappointment that accompany a PCOS diagnosis. My goal is to show afflicted women that they can restore their fertility, conquer their embarrassing acne and male-pattern hair growth, and lead happier, low-stress lives. This book describes how PCOS and insulin resistance develop in women, and it presents a number of diet, exercise, and lifestyle guidelines that can dramatically improve your symptoms and quality of life.

PCOS is a common condition that can be managed effectively, once you learn how. I promise that you are not alone on this journey and, no matter how bad things might feel, there is light at the end of the tunnel!

Jennifer's Story

The first things I want you to know are that you *can* regain control of your health and that you are not alone. During my sixteen years of practice as a registered dietitian nutritionist, I have worked with many women diagnosed with PCOS, who come to me frustrated with their health issues and confused about the proper dietary approach they should take. I start by educating my clients on the components of a healthy diet for PCOS, and then I emphasize mini-goals, such as maintaining a current weight rather than losing weight—which is difficult for those who have PCOS. Together we develop a workable meal plan for reducing insulin levels by focusing on foods that reverse insulin resistance, reduce cardiovascular risk factors, improve fertility, and assist in weight loss. It is with these goals in mind that I created the recipes in this book.

The recipes in this book include foods that have unique nutritional profiles beneficial for women with PCOS. Chronic inflammation underlies most metabolic disorders, so you will see an emphasis on key anti-inflammatory, slow burning, low glycemic index carbs like quinoa, millet, rolled oats, brown rice, beans, vegetables, and whole fruits; lean protein sources including fish, chicken, lean beef, eggs, soy foods, low-fat or nonfat dairy products, legumes, nuts, and seeds; and healthy fats from foods like avocado, nuts, seeds, and olives. All culinary herbs and spices have antioxidants, too, but these have the most: basil, cloves, oregano, rosemary, cinnamon, turmeric, and sage. You will see them used often in the recipes.

Weight management concerns will be addressed in the recipes through the use of ingredients that promote satiety, the feeling of fullness, and reduce cravings for other unhealthy choices. The recipe label "lower calorie" makes it easy to quickly find recipes that are appropriate for managing your weight. Throughout the book, recipes will also include tips for making substitutions or additions to lower the calorie count or include a nutrient shown to assist in weight management.

While all of the recipes in this book are appropriate for women with PCOS trying to conceive, recipes with the "fertility boost" designation are particularly high in nutrients known to naturally increase fertility. Your preconception diet should have an emphasis on low glycemic index carbohydrates, and should include less meat and more plant proteins, ample omega-3 fats, and antioxidant-rich foods that are high in vitamins C, E, D; folate; and carotenoids, as well as minerals like selenium, zinc, and copper.

Also in this book (in chapter 2), I have included a day-by-day, four-week meal plan to help you get started on the diet. I've also provided shopping guides to pantry staples and essential cooking equipment, which list groceries and tools you will need to make the recipes.

The diet outlined in this book is more about what you can eat, rather than what you cannot eat. I encourage you to enjoy discovering the variety of flavors and textures that await you.

I The PCOS Diet Plan

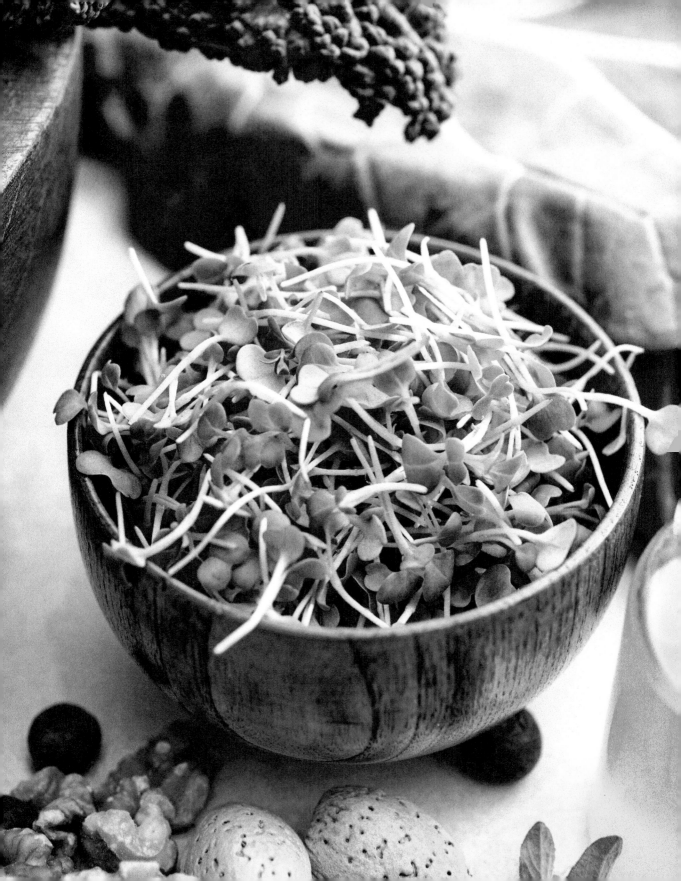

1

Insulin Resistance and PCOS

Polycystic ovarian syndrome (PCOS) is a common condition that affects about 10 percent of the female population in the Western world (Dunaif, 1997). It is the leading cause of infertility in these women, and if left untreated, it can increase their risk of developing endometrial cancer. Although PCOS cannot be completely cured, its symptoms can be managed. The most important symptom to treat is insulin resistance because of its associated effects on androgens—the hormones that are produced in excessive amounts in women with PCOS and directly affect normal reproductive functioning. Overcoming insulin resistance has a positive carryover effect on other PCOS symptoms, such as infertility, acne, and mood swings.

At least 50 percent of women with PCOS are insulin resistant, and around 10 percent of all women who are insulin resistant suffer from PCOS (Dunaif, 1997). The close relationship between PCOS and insulin resistance is more prevalent in obese women with PCOS: about 80 percent will develop insulin resistance by the age of 40 (Healthy Women, 2015).

Although plenty of documented research exists on insulin resistance (we have recommended our favorite books, organizations, and websites in the Resources section at the back of this book), less information is available on how insulin resistance can be managed while dealing with the additional challenges of PCOS.

This chapter describes the basics of metabolic function and the causes and symptoms of PCOS, as well as the link between PCOS and insulin resistance, and then discusses in detail the Insulin Resistance Diet for PCOS and the short- and long-term effects you can expect to experience while following the plan.

Always consult your doctor before making any major dietary or lifestyle changes, including the program discussed in this book.

Metabolism in Women

The metabolism of a normal, healthy person is responsible for extracting energy from what the person eats and drinks in order to sustain life, which includes everything from moving and breathing to growing and repairing cells. Metabolism involves a series of chemical reactions that both store and convert molecules into energy. Although everyone has a metabolism, metabolic efficiency can vary from person to person based on a number of factors.

What most people refer to when they speak about their metabolism (e.g., by stating that their metabolism is slower than it used to be) is actually their basal metabolic rate (BMR). Your BMR is the amount of energy your body requires to maintain daily life, and it is expressed as the number of calories per day you burn at rest if you are completely sedentary. The average BMR in the United States is 1,493 calories for women and 1,662 calories for men (Hutchinson, 2014). Your total energy expenditure per day also includes the amount of calories you burn during exercise and incidental activity, as well as the heat-producing act of simply digesting and metabolizing your food.

Your BMR is affected by your age, sex, genetics, height, and weight. It can be slowed down during an extended period of restricted caloric intake; so for that reason, it is important to consistently eat an amount of calories that are approximately equal to your BMR. Conversely, your BMR can be sped up by increasing lean muscle tissue (e.g., through resistance training, obtaining an adequate amount of sleep, and reducing stress levels).

Upon reaching adulthood, women tend to lose around 150 calories from their BMR with each decade (Roberts and Dallal, 2005). This occurs as your production of human growth hormone drops, activity levels tend to slow down with age, and highly metabolically active muscle mass is lost while relatively metabolically inactive fat tissue is gained.

This reduction in your BMR can be slowed by doing resistance training two or three times a week to prevent muscle atrophy and boost human growth hormone production. There is no reason why a woman who was sedentary throughout her twenties and thirties cannot have a higher metabolic rate in her forties if she changes her exercise regime. (You'll find more information about the ideal exercise routine for PCOS on page 29.)

The most significant hormone involved in the metabolism process is insulin, which is produced by the pancreas. Insulin is responsible for regulating the level of glucose in your blood, and it also enables your cells to take in glucose, which may be used immediately for energy or stored for later use. In healthy individuals, insulin is released in small doses throughout the day, with extra amounts produced at mealtimes.

The Role of Food

The foods we consume directly affect our metabolism and insulin response. All food is made up of three macronutrients in varying quantities: protein, fat, and carbohydrates. Each macronutrient plays a crucial role in normal body functioning and affects our metabolism differently.

Protein is responsible for the growth and repair of body tissue, and it is occasionally used as an energy source. The best sources of protein are lean meats, fish, poultry, eggs, and legumes.

Fat protects our internal organs, regulates body temperature, processes vitamins, and also repairs body tissue. For optimal health, eat monounsaturated fats (e.g., olive, canola, peanut, safflower, and sesame oils; avocados; and nuts and seeds) and polyunsaturated fats (e.g., soybean, corn, and sunflower oils; fatty fish; walnuts; sunflower seeds; and soybeans and tofu). Avoid saturated fats (mostly found in animal sources of food, such as red meats, poultry with skin, and full-fat dairy) and trans fats (found in processed foods and snack foods such as chips and crackers).

Carbohydrates are the body's preferred source of energy, because they do not need to be converted before use, unlike protein or fat. Simple carbohydrates—as found in cookies, chocolate, fruit, soda, white rice, and white flour products—are quickly digested sources of energy. Because these foods cause sudden increases and drops in blood sugar levels, they should be avoided by insulin-resistant individuals. Instead, fill your carbohydrate needs with slow-digesting, complex forms of carbohydrates, such as beans, oatmeal, potatoes, brown rice, and whole wheat flour products.

Although insulin-resistant individuals have a poor tolerance of carbohydrates, relative to the two other macronutrients (since carbohydrates are broken down into glucose, and consequently must be managed by the individual's poorly functioning insulin response), carbohydrates still play a crucial role in maintaining a healthy metabolism. You should therefore consume complex, unprocessed forms of carbohydrates in your diet while you are attempting to overcome your insulin resistance.

Ensuring that your diet is made up of healthy proteins, complex carbohydrates, and mono- and polyunsaturated fats will help control the release of insulin and foster a healthy metabolism, even if yours has functioned poorly in the past.

Insulin Resistance

A malfunction in the metabolic process can lead to insulin resistance. This occurs either when the body does not produce enough insulin to meet its needs or when the cells build up a resistance to insulin. Although there may be insulin present in the bloodstream, the amount is not enough to trigger the uptake of nutrients by the cells. While the body subsequently demands more insulin, glucose may build up in the bloodstream. Then, when glucose is finally taken into the cells, some insulin is left over in the bloodstream because too much has been released during this process. These factors combined cause the beta cells of the pancreas to malfunction and, in turn, cause your body to become less and less sensitive to the demands of insulin. Over time, insulin resistance can lead to weight gain and the development of diabetes.

Insulin resistance can develop as a result of a nutrient-poor diet high in refined carbohydrates, but it can also occur as a result of low-carbohydrate crash diets and excessive amounts of exercise—both of which can create stress within the body, shut down normal hormone production, and trigger polycystic ovarian syndrome.

PCOS Basics

A woman with a healthy reproductive system has ovaries that produce eggs and fallopian tubes that carry a fertilized egg from the ovaries to the uterus, where the egg can continue to develop as a fetus within the thickened uterine lining. If fertilization does not occur, the uterine lining is shed in a process known as menstruation. This cycle of events lasts about 28 days in a healthy woman and is governed by the production of four key hormones: follicle-stimulating hormone, luteinizing hormone, estrogen, and progesterone. The amounts of these hormones must maintain a delicate balance to function correctly.

One thing that can interfere with the natural function of these hormones is androgens. Androgens are known as "male hormones"; however, they are present in the bodies of both men and women, in varying degrees. Although a healthy woman produces only around 5 to 10 percent of the androgens produced by her male counterpart (Healthy Line, 2015), her body is more sensitive to their effects. The three principal androgens are testosterone, dihydrotestosterone, and androstenedione. They regulate the function of many organs, synthesize estrogen, and prevent bone loss.

PCOS is characterized by multiple cysts on the ovaries, an irregular or absent menstrual cycle, infertility, blood sugar disorders (such as insulin resistance), and elevated levels of androgens, which can cause acne, facial hair, mood swings, and excess weight gain, as well as increased difficulty in losing weight. While some women may unfortunately be inflicted with all of these symptoms, most exhibit only a few. And, contrary to what the name itself suggests, not all women with PCOS have polycystic ovaries. Some women do not exhibit any symptoms at all and only discover that they have PCOS when they find it difficult to conceive.

PCOS is usually diagnosed by an ultrasound, which confirms the presence of cysts, and blood tests, which demonstrate the type of hormonal imbalance that exists.

Unlike during the normal reproductive process, where an egg is released each month, the egg in women with PCOS either does not develop or is not released during ovulation. This situation is primarily the result of elevated levels of androgens, which also cause cysts to form and menstrual cycles to become irregular. If left untreated, these hormone imbalances can create serious long-term consequences, such as insulin resistance and diabetes, high cholesterol, high blood pressure, heart disease, depression, sleep apnea, and endometrial

cancer. Women with PCOS typically require close monitoring during pregnancy because of their higher risk for miscarriage, gestational diabetes, and premature delivery.

A multitude of factors can cause PCOS. While every case is different and the reasons for that are not all well understood by the medical community, what is clear is that PCOS is linked to a hormonal imbalance. A change in one hormone causes a change in another, which then affects another, and so on, thereby altering the complicated reproductive cycle.

The most common cause of PCOS is insulin resistance, which is usually linked to a poor diet and being overweight. PCOS is sometimes triggered when your reproductive organs undergo a period of significant stress, which includes not only psychological stress but also the stress of being underweight, dieting for too long, or exercising in excessive amounts. Genetics also play a role in developing PCOS: for example, if your mother or sister has the condition, you are more likely to be predisposed to it.

In some cases, the signs of PCOS crop up immediately after a teenage girl starts menstruating. In other cases, PCOS functions as an underlying genetic condition that is triggered by certain environmental stimuli later in a woman's life, such as specific foods (particularly sugar, soy, gluten, and dairy), lifestyle behaviors, or high levels of stress.

Although PCOS cannot be cured, its symptoms can be managed through diet and lifestyle changes so that its sufferers can live normal, happy lives. Learning to control your PCOS will lower your risk of infertility, miscarriage, diabetes, and heart disease. While medical treatment will vary from woman to woman, all women will benefit from following a healthy diet and taking up a regular exercise regime.

In addition to lifestyle changes, your doctor may also recommend certain medications to manage your PCOS and insulin resistance. The birth control pill is often prescribed to women who do not wish to become pregnant, since it helps regulate their cycles and lower the levels of androgens in their bodies. The birth control pill, though, does not address the underlying cause of PCOS, and women may experience even greater hormonal dysfunctions when they stop taking it. Women who have PCOS and want to become pregnant are often given fertility drugs, such as clomiphene, to assist in ovulation. It is still possible to get pregnant and have a healthy birth with PCOS.

Anti-androgen medicines, such as spironolactone and flutamide, block the effects of androgens, which can help control superficial symptoms of PCOS like acne and hair growth. Topical medications can also assist in reducing these symptoms. Diabetes medications, such as metformin, are also commonly prescribed to lower blood glucose and testosterone levels. And these medications can, in turn, assist in ovulation, stimulate a regular menstrual cycle, and encourage weight loss.

For Tara, her PCOS went undiscovered until she came off the birth control pill after being on it for six years and then did not menstruate for 18 months afterward. After giving her the diagnosis, Tara's doctor suggested that she simply go back on the pill. Tara chose not to, since she believed that relying on artificial hormones once again would only mask the underlying problem. Instead, she sought out natural treatment methods to manage her PCOS symptoms, with great success.

The Link Between PCOS and Insulin Resistance

A recent study (Stepto et al., 2013) found that 95 percent of overweight women with PCOS and 75 percent of lean women with PCOS were also insulin resistant. The connection is primarily caused by abnormally high insulin levels in the blood stimulating excessive production of testosterone in the ovaries, which results in PCOS (Nestler et al., 1998). But the connection can go both ways: Androgens can also act directly on peripheral tissues to reduce insulin receptor sensitivity and create defects in the movements of glucose transporters, which promotes insulin resistance (Livingstone and Collison, 2002).

Many women with PCOS also suffer from low-grade inflammation, whereby the white blood cells of the body swarm to a perceived internal threat that does not actually require an inflammatory response. This process causes the cells to start attacking internal organs and tissues, and can cause insulin resistance. It is usually caused by eating certain foods or being exposed to particular environmental factors such as toxins, stress, or inadequate sleep.

Even if your body's levels of follicle-stimulating hormone, luteinizing hormone, estrogen, and progesterone are normal, normal menstruation will not occur if testosterone levels are high. It is therefore imperative to learn how to normalize your insulin levels in order to reduce androgen production, since doing so will simultaneously address a host of other issues.

Overcoming insulin resistance can help restore fertility, reverse an irregular menstrual cycle, promote weight loss, and overcome the male-pattern symptoms of PCOS, such as acne, baldness, and excess hair growth. It will also prevent the development of future complications, such as metabolic syndrome, cardiac problems, or type 2 diabetes. More than 50 percent of women with PCOS develop prediabetes and diabetes before the age of 40 (Women's Health, 2016).

Reducing circulating levels of insulin in the bloodstream often leads to weight loss, which should be encouraged for overweight women with PCOS. As little as a 5 to 7 percent reduction in body weight over a six-month period can lower insulin and androgen levels, consequently restoring ovulation and fertility in more than 75 percent of obese PCOS women (Kiddy et al., 1992).

However, not all women who suffer from PCOS and insulin resistance are overweight. Instead of focusing on weight loss, these women should simply stick to a healthy, low-glycemic diet, exercise regularly, and manage their stress levels in order to nurture their bodies back to full health.

Insulin plays an extremely important role in a healthy metabolism and normal body functioning, so it is crucial that it functions properly. Even the simple fact of knowing that insulin resistance can be overcome—unlike PCOS itself—can do wonders for gaining self-confidence and finding the motivation to stick to a healthy diet and exercise plan.

For Tara, overcoming her insulin resistance was the best thing she did for her PCOS. Once she accomplished that, her stubborn acne finally began to fade; she experienced a regular menstrual cycle for the first time in her life; her metabolism stabilized, allowing her to finally enjoy carbohydrates in abundance; and she lost the weight around her midsection, which had been persisting for years.

Although some medical professionals dismissed the connection in the past, more practitioners are now recommending a healthy diet as part of a PCOS treatment plan. Doctors are increasingly recognizing the importance of treating one of the underlying causes of PCOS—insulin resistance—rather than tackling each of the symptoms individually. Consequently, there is an increasing shift toward natural treatment methods, which can stimulate a number of positive benefits without the negative side effects triggered by many common drugs.

TARA'S ADVICE FOR THE NEWLY DIAGNOSED

When I received my PCOS diagnosis, I was devastated. Even though I instinctively knew that something was not right with my hormones and reproductive system—because I'd never had a regular menstrual cycle, I found it extremely difficult to lose weight, and I was suffering worse acne in my twenties than I had in my teen years—the diagnosis still came as a shock.

I was worried that I would never be able to have children, and that I would be doomed to a life of restricting carbohydrate intake in order to manage my insulin resistance.

Most heartbreakingly, I felt isolated, because none of my friends had this condition.

Here are seven pieces of advice that I wish I'd been given at the beginning of my PCOS journey:

Track your PCOS symptoms: Keep a record of your menstrual cycle (duration of menstruation and time between cycles, level of flow, and severity of symptoms) and other PCOS-related symptoms, such as acne, hair growth, and changes in body weight. This information will assist you in discovering the direct relationship between your PCOS and any dietary and lifestyle changes you implement.

Keep a food diary: As you will come to learn in the next section of this chapter, what you eat and drink has a direct impact on your hormonal health. After you eat certain foods, you may notice that your symptoms worsen or your menstruation cycle is delayed. A diary will enable you to identify your trigger foods.

Realize that having PCOS does not mean you are infertile: One of the biggest fears for women with PCOS is that they will never be able to conceive. Many affected women are able to become pregnant naturally—or if not, with the help of fertility drugs—and go on to have healthy pregnancies and births. It just may take a little longer than for the average woman.

Accept that your PCOS will require some lifestyle changes: Although PCOS is an underlying medical condition and therefore not something you can blame yourself for having, certain lifestyle choices can worsen your symptoms. You must be honest with yourself in acknowledging what may be causing your particular case of PCOS, and make the necessary dietary and lifestyle changes. The sooner you accept this, the faster you will be able to heal.

Do not be afraid to seek further medical guidance: While your doctor will be able to inform you about the basic options available for managing your PCOS, you might also consider seeing an endocrinologist who specializes in hormonal health, an alternative practitioner such as an acupuncturist, or a therapist to deal with the emotional ramifications of your diagnosis.

Connect with other women: The one good thing about PCOS is that it is a very common condition. Even if you do not personally know anyone who has it, you can connect with thousands of women online who do (I have listed my favorite forums in the Resources section on page 209). There is no need to ever feel alone during this difficult journey.

Be patient: Overcoming insulin resistance and successfully managing PCOS are not things that happen overnight. Every woman is different and will require a slightly different plan of attack to heal her body, which may involve a long period of experimentation. Once you discover the underlying cause of your PCOS and take steps to overcome it, you must give your body adequate time to heal.

The Insulin Resistance Diet for PCOS

Overcoming your insulin resistance must be the first step you take toward managing your PCOS. Given that your hormonal health is closely linked to the foods you eat, the bulk of the changes required are dietary.

To restore your insulin sensitivity and manage PCOS, you must eliminate processed foods, which are often full of toxins and chemicals. Instead, nourish your body with nutrient-dense whole foods that are as close to their natural state as possible, such as lean meats, fresh fruits and vegetables, and high-fiber whole grains, nuts, and seeds. These natural foods will promote and support a proper hormonal balance and a strong metabolism.

Keep the following guidelines in mind when complying with the Insulin Resistance Diet for PCOS.

Avoid sugar, soy, dairy, trans fats, and artificial sweeteners. Sugar clearly has the largest impact on insulin, but it also increases cravings, leads to overeating, and plays a strong role in obesity. Soy is a phytoestrogen, meaning that it resembles natural estrogen within the body and therefore impedes its natural production. Both gluten and dairy can cause inflammation in the body and may also cause poor gut health and insulin resistance. In addition, dairy products tend to be highly processed and highly hormonal foods. Trans fats also cause inflammation and metabolic distress, which can lead to fat storage and insulin resistance over time. Although artificial sweeteners do not contain sugar and therefore do not increase blood glucose levels, they still stimulate the release of insulin and fuel cravings for sugar.

Do not eliminate carbohydrates completely. Although your body may not tolerate carbohydrates well, it is important to consume complex, high-fiber forms—such as legumes, quinoa, brown rice, buckwheat, millet, and vegetables—to improve your insulin sensitivity. Avoid refined, processed types of carbohydrates, such as refined sugars, white flour, and white rice.

Consume carbohydrates that are low on the glycemic index. The glycemic index rates foods from 0 to 100, based on how the food affects a person's blood glucose level. Low-glycemic foods (with a rating of 55 or less) cause a slow release of glucose into your bloodstream. High-glycemic foods (with a rating of 70 or above) increase your blood sugar levels faster, stimulating a greater amount of insulin secretion and, in turn, possibly increasing insulin resistance and body fat levels. For a full list of common carbohydrates on the glycemic index, see Appendix A on page 201. Lower glycemic foods also typically contain more fiber than higher glycemic foods, which helps increase satiety, further reduces the rate of insulin release, and promotes healthy estrogen metabolism.

Consume carbohydrates with low glycemic loads. You must also pay attention to the glycemic load of a food, or the amount of carbohydrates the food contains per serving. Some foods, such as carrots and watermelon, are high on the glycemic index, but would have to be eaten in extremely large quantities to carry a high glycemic load. Therefore, it is often more useful to consider the glycemic load rather than the glycemic index of a particular food when deciding if it fits into your diet. All of the foods in the Foods to Enjoy table on page 23 have a low glycemic load.

Eat three main meals and two snacks per day. Although it is important to keep blood sugar levels stable throughout the day by eating every three to four hours, avoid continually snacking, since it interferes with the normal signaling and functioning of insulin and other hormones.

All meals should contain a mix of lean proteins, complex carbohydrates, and healthy fats. To avoid spikes in blood sugar from eating too many carbohydrates at a time, space your carbohydrates out evenly throughout most—if not all—of your meals during the day. Do not eat carbohydrates by themselves; always combine them with protein and/or fat to encourage a more gradual release of energy. Vegetables are rich in vitamins and antioxidants and should be eaten at every meal, while fruit should be limited to one or two servings per day.

Around 40 to 50 percent of your daily caloric intake should come from carbohydrates. Women who have PCOS but are not overweight should set their carbohydrate intake to less than half of their daily caloric intake (at least 100 grams of carbohydrates per day). Women who have PCOS and are overweight should limit their carbohydrate intake to less than 40 percent of their daily intake. Protein should be set at an equal amount to carbohydrates (40 percent), with healthy fats like avocados, fatty fish, olive oil, and nuts making up the balance (20 percent).

Choose organic sources of protein where possible. Recommended sources of protein include lean meats, fish, poultry, eggs, and legumes. Conventionally raised animals are typically pumped full of estrogen and antibiotics, which can negatively affect human hormones. So it is best to choose meat products from organic, grass-fed animals.

Stick to water and noncaffeinated herbal teas. As caffeine has been shown to increase insulin resistance by about 15 percent (Biaggioni and Davis, 2002), it should be avoided. Alcohol should also be avoided, since it is highly inflammatory, it is metabolized as a toxin, and it is also likely to inspire less than ideal food choices.

Consider supplementation. Alongside a natural diet, certain supplements have been shown to promote optimal hormonal health and natural ovulation. These include calcium, chromium, co-enzyme Q10, cod liver oil, diindolylmethane (DIM), evening primrose oil, gymnema, iodine, magnesium, N-acetyl cysteine, selenium, taurine, vitamin B_6, vitamin D, and zinc. Among the naturally derived supplements on the market, vitex agnus-castus, apple cider vinegar, cinnamon, fenugreek, flaxseed, licorice root, maca, milk thistle, saw palmetto, and spearmint tea are particularly beneficial for women with PCOS. I've personally seen the best results from vitex agnus-castus, DIM, and magnesium. For more information about supplements, please see the Resources section on page 209.

The principles of this diet will help you lose weight naturally if you are overweight, and you can expect further weight loss once your hormonal system starts to heal. Keep in mind that weight loss is very important to managing PCOS, since just a 5 to 7 percent loss in total bodyweight can restore fertility. You can deliberately reduce your caloric intake to speed up the weight loss process, but never drop below around 1,500 calories per day, because that will create additional hormonal stress within your body.

Even if you are not overweight, it is important to avoid gaining weight during this process. Following the Insulin Resistance Diet for PCOS will ensure you do not.

This diet is meant to address all of the different symptoms associated with PCOS. However, if you wish to focus on your own personal goals, such as trying to conceive, losing weight, or lowering inflammation, simply choose recipes from part 2 of this book that are labeled "Fertility Boost," "Lower Calorie," or "Inflammation Fighter."

Adhere to the recommendations in the following table, and you will be well on your way to overcoming your insulin resistance and conquering your PCOS.

Setting Reasonable Expectations

If you are completely overhauling your lifestyle and switching from a standard American diet filled with inflammatory and toxic foods, you may see benefits immediately after commencing the Insulin Resistance Diet for PCOS. For those who are already following a relatively healthy diet, or are dealing with the added problem of stress, it may take a bit longer for you to see positive results.

During the recovery process, you may experience both positive and negative side effects as your body goes through its recovery. It is important to be aware of this, and to remind yourself that the longstanding positives of the process far outweigh the fleeting negatives. These effects can vary from cravings, headaches, and reduced energy levels in the short term, to a regular menstrual cycle, weight loss, improved fertility, and improved insulin sensitivity in the long term.

Although the process can sometimes feel daunting, remind yourself that conquering the short-term discomforts will set you up

FOODS TO ENJOY AND FOODS TO AVOID

FOODS TO ENJOY

Fish (cod, halibut, herring, salmon, sardines)

Lean meats (organic, pasture-raised beef, lamb, and pork; chicken and turkey)

Eggs

Legumes (black beans, chickpeas, lentils, soybeans)

Low-glycemic index vegetables (asparagus, broccoli, Brussels sprouts, cabbage, kale, spinach)

Low-glycemic index fruits (apples, berries, cherries, peaches, pears, plums, rhubarb)

Medium-glycemic index fruits (cantaloupes, grapes, kiwifruit)

Whole grains (amaranth, buckwheat, millet, quinoa, teff)

Extra-virgin olive oil, coconut oil, flaxseed oil

Nuts and seeds (almonds, flaxseed, macadamia nuts, pumpkin seeds, walnuts)

Garlic

Dairy alternatives (almond, coconut, and hazelnut milks)

Dark chocolate

FOODS TO AVOID

Alcohol

All foods containing white sugar and flour (bagels, breads, cereals, pasta, pastries)

All foods containing high-fructose corn syrup (breakfast cereals, juices, ketchup, salad dressings, soda)

All foods containing hydrogenated oils (cakes, candy, chips, doughnuts)

Artificial sweeteners (acesulfame potassium, aspartame, saccharin, sorbitol)

Fish containing mercury (shark, swordfish, tuna, tilefish)

High-glycemic index vegetables (corn, rutabagas, parsnips, potatoes, turnips)

Most dairy

Processed fruit juices

Processed oils (canola, corn, peanut, safflower, sunflower)

Red meat (unless organic or pasture-raised) and organ meats

for long-term success. Although the journey requires patience, experimentation, and self-discovery, your body is clever and will begin to heal once you point it in the right direction.

What to Expect in the Short Term

Your body may respond negatively when it is initially deprived of processed foods, and the more processed your diet was originally, the more severe your negative symptoms may be. These symptoms will typically last anywhere from one to two weeks before they, fortunately, pave the way for the positive, long-term side effects of the diet to take place.

Cravings and Headaches
Processed foods common in the standard American diet contain addictive properties, meaning that you will likely experience headaches and strong cravings for the foods you initially cut out of your diet. Once these toxins have been completely removed from your bloodstream, you will no longer crave them. Do not keep any processed foods in the house; instead, keep healthy snacks nearby for when cravings strike.

Varying Energy Levels
Some people may initially feel more lethargic after commencing this diet, as their bodies detox from high-calorie processed foods. Others, however, may immediately feel more energetic once they begin to eat healthier, more nutritious foods. Ultimately, everyone will end up with higher energy levels and better sleep quality compared to when they began the diet.

Weight Loss
It is common to lose weight almost immediately after beginning this diet, particularly if you combine it with the exercise recommendations in chapter 2. This is because you will almost certainly be eating fewer calories than before, as well as fewer foods that encourage fat storage among insulin-resistant individuals. The exact amount and rate of weight loss will depend on how poor your nutritional intake was before starting this diet.

Weight loss should happen naturally and almost effortlessly, and will continue into the future as your insulin sensitivity continues to improve. Even mild weight loss can have an extremely positive carryover effect on your PCOS symptoms, since it immediately reduces the production of male hormones in the body and encourages ovulation to occur naturally.

What to Expect in the Long Term

All of the long-term effects of following this diet are positive. It is important, though, to commit to your new dietary and lifestyle changes for at least six months before expecting to see any major improvements in your PCOS symptoms.

Better Digestion

Foods containing dairy, gluten, and sugar negatively affect your digestive system. By minimizing your intake of these foods, you will see a reduction in bloating, constipation, and diarrhea, if applicable, and you will experience more regular bowel movements.

Decreased Cravings

Although you may initially experience strong cravings for processed foods, these will lessen over time. The longer you stick with the diet, the easier it will become. Your desire to eat unhealthy foods will become less and less as you see how well your body responds to a natural, whole foods–based diet. You may be surprised to even find yourself craving fresh fruits and vegetables!

Fewer Ovarian Cysts

By improving your hormonal health, you will reduce the number of cysts on your ovaries (if applicable) and, in turn, reduced the amount of associated abdominal pain.

Improved Moods

Mood swings are a common symptom of PCOS, which can be exacerbated by high-carbohydrate and high-fat foods that trigger blood sugar spikes and drops. By basing your diet on foods that keep your blood sugar levels steady, you will experience fewer mood swings and an improvement in concentration.

Increased Fertility

Most important, this diet will help you restore your fertility by improving the signaling between the pituitary gland and the ovaries. This will increase your chances of natural ovulation and conception, improve the condition of the uterus for implantation, and reduce the risk of miscarriage as well as the development of diabetes from insulin resistance (Natural Fertility Info, 2016).

Increased Insulin Sensitivity

This diet will help you overcome insulin resistance, which will reduce your body's androgen production and support proper reproductive health.

Reduced Blood Pressure

When you improve your diet overall and eat less sugar and saturated and trans fats, your blood pressure will drop. This will, in turn, decrease your risk of heart attack, heart disease, stroke, and other diseases (American Heart Association, 2015).

Reduced Inflammation

By eliminating highly inflammatory foods like dairy, gluten, and soy, you will reduce inflammation and thereby improve your immunity.

Reduced Male-Pattern Symptoms

Improved insulin sensitivity and reduced androgen production will cause male-associated PCOS symptoms (acne, hair growth, and baldness) to lessen. Tara's worst PCOS symptom is acne, and she has been able to manage it better by making diet changes—particularly avoiding dairy and sugar—than by taking any medication.

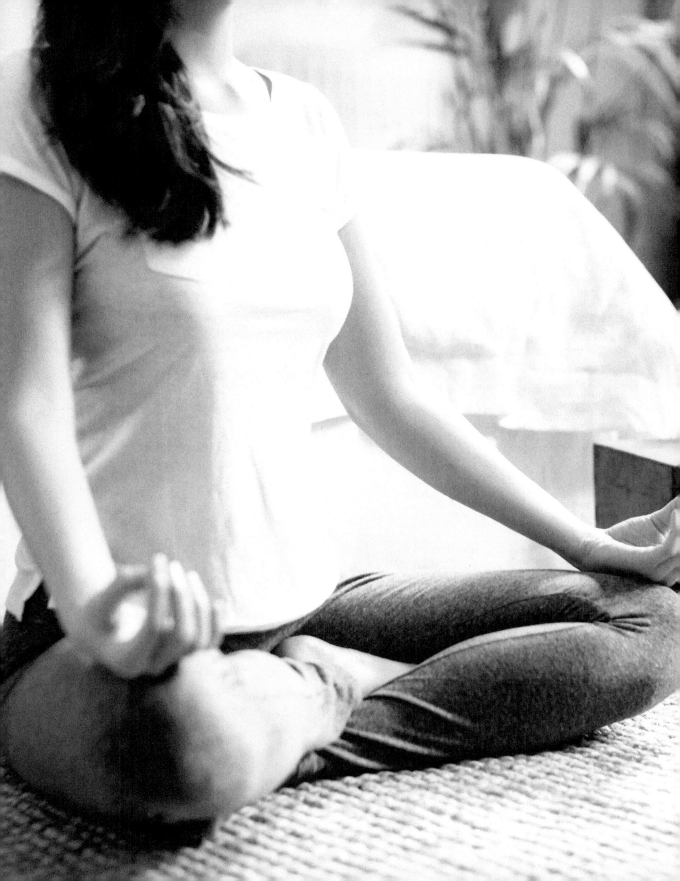

2

Living Well to Eat Well

Although following the principles of the Insulin Resistance Diet for PCOS will help you overcome your insulin resistance, a host of additional physical and emotional factors must also be considered in your journey to achieving full hormonal health.

This chapter teaches you how to improve your health through lifestyle changes and provides tips for treating your body with kindness and love, which is crucial during this challenging period.

The Importance of a Healthy Lifestyle

Because of the effects of the following factors on insulin, cortisol, and androgen production, it is crucial to address each one when attempting to overcome your PCOS, especially if you are trying to conceive.

Your guiding principle throughout this journey should be to move toward natural nourishment. This means not only eating whole foods that will optimize your health, but also learning to prioritize your sleep, reduce stress, and exercise regularly.

Rest and Sleep

Sleep is critical for optimal metabolic function and insulin sensitivity, since the body's hormonal production peaks during sleep. Poor sleep patterns may increase your overall appetite and calorie consumption, as well as the rate of fat storage in your body (Kondracki, 2012). Regularly getting a good night's sleep is also important for the health of your skin, cognitive function, and athletic performance.

In general, it is important to take time to rest and relax, particularly if you have a highly stressful life. Unwinding for 30 to 60 minutes a day goes hand-in-hand with maintaining good sleep habits.

To improve the quality of your sleep, try the following tips.

Sleep between seven and nine hours a night, in a completely dark, quiet, and cool room. Use heavy curtains or blackout shades to block all light, or wear a sleep mask. To block outside noise, wear earplugs or use a sound machine. The ideal temperature for sleeping is around 65 degrees Fahrenheit.

Go to sleep and wake up at the same time every day. Ensure that you have a regular sleep-wake cycle, or circadian rhythm, because this will optimize the quality of your sleep. Going to sleep when you naturally feel tired should enable you to wake naturally without an alarm clock. Sadly, "catching up" on sleep on the weekend does not work (Cohen et al., 2010).

Turn off all electronics at least one hour before bed. The bright lights emitted from your phone, tablet, computer, or television prevent your body from falling into a deep sleep, because your body will still think it is daylight outside. If you must use a computer in the evening, use the light-dimming function. Before you go to sleep, do something restful and relaxing such as reading, listening to music, meditating, or spending time with a loved one.

Exercise regularly. Exercise will improve your energy levels throughout the day and make it easier to fall asleep at night. But avoid exercising within three hours of bedtime.

Do not consume caffeine six to eight hours before bedtime. You should avoid coffee, tea, chocolate, and energy drinks, as well as other stimulants like nicotine and alcohol, in the afternoon hours before sleep.

Reserve your bed for sleep only. Do not watch television or bring your laptop into your bed, for example, because you will have a harder time switching off your brain at the end of the day. Keep a piece of paper next to your bed to jot down any thoughts that enter your mind in the night, and then try not to think about them until morning.

Pleasure and Joy

Stress management plays an extremely important role in the natural treatment of your PCOS symptoms. There are two main types of stress: physical stress caused by overexercising, undereating, or eating foods filled with toxins; and psychological stress caused by family or relationship problems, work-related anxiety, or the general demands of hectic modern life. The two types are nearly indistinguishable within the brain, and both increase adrenal function, which, in turn, increases cortisol secretion, elevates blood sugar levels, and increases insulin and androgen production. Stress also exacerbates internal inflammation, affects proper immune system function, and even damages brain chemistry (Chetty et al., 2014).

All of these factors combined signal to the body that it is not a good time to reproduce, and in response, your menstrual cycle is suspended. To manage PCOS, it is imperative to reduce psychological stress. Try the following tips:

Perform at least one stress-relieving activity per day. This may include meditation, yoga, reading, taking a warm bath, spending time with friends, or therapy. A good time to do this is right before bed, as relaxation will improve your quality of sleep.

Cease activities that cause stress. For example, avoid undereating, fasting, over-exercising, and undersleeping.

Do not treat relaxation activities as merely an option for when you have the time. Instead, prioritize them as an essential part of your daily life to keep your mind and body healthy.

Use resources for guidance. There are plenty of mobile applications, audio recordings on Amazon, and instructional videos on YouTube that will guide you through meditation or yoga. You can also use Meetup.com to find relaxation-focused groups. These groups are often free, or at least much cheaper than professional options.

Physical Activity

Exercise and ordinary physical activity allow your body to maintain a proper hormonal balance and a regular metabolic function, by increasing the rate of glucose uptake by muscle cells (Colberg et al., 2010). Partaking in a regular exercise program will also help control your weight, which is an important part of overcoming insulin resistance.

Even if you do not lose weight, don't underestimate the impact of regular exercise on your hormonal and metabolic health. A recent study (Hutchinson et al., 2011) found that women who performed just three hours of aerobic exercise per week over a 12-week period improved their insulin sensitivity and lost visceral fat, despite not losing weight.

It can sometimes be difficult to find the time and motivation to exercise. Here are five tips to keep you on track:

Remind yourself of the benefits of physical activity. Strength training will improve your metabolism by building metabolically active muscle tissue, while aerobic exercise sharpens insulin sensitivity and lowers blood sugar levels.

Find a form of exercise that you enjoy and can look forward to. This type of exercise might be decompressing in a power yoga class, taking the family on a nature hike, swimming in the ocean, bicycling along a pleasant nature trail, or shaking your booty in a Zumba class. Participating in enjoyable exercise will lower your stress levels, too.

Exercise for at least 30 minutes per day, at least five days a week. Your workouts may involve resistance machines and free weights, your own body weight, or moderate-intensity aerobic exercise. You can find many free workout programs online, but you may also consider hiring a personal trainer to learn correct form.

Exercise a moderate amount at a moderate intensity. It is important to avoid excessive, high-intensity exercise programs, because they will trigger the release of cortisol, increase inflammation, and consequently make your PCOS worse. Throwing yourself into an intense exercise regime often backfires by overworking your adrenal glands and making fat loss more difficult. To ensure proper recovery, take at least one or two full rest days per week.

Prioritize your health, and treat your workouts like any other important appointment. Keep your gym bag in your car ready for when you finish work, invest in some hand weights and resistance bands for home or office breaks, or take a walk in the fresh air during your lunch break.

The Power of Healthy Habits

The thought of changing your diet, starting a new exercise regime, and making time for self-care and stress-relieving activities may seem overwhelming, and you may not know where to begin. Start by setting small, realistic goals and tackling one at a time.

The key to being successful is sticking to your goals. This may involve creating a brand new habit, but it will most often involve replacing a bad habit with a good one. For example, you may have a daily habit of hitting up the office vending machine for a candy bar during your mid-afternoon slump. Instead, pack a healthy snack, such as an apple and a handful of nuts. In the evenings, your bad habit might involve collapsing onto the sofa with a bag of potato chips in hand. Swap the potato chips for some boxing gloves and try out a local class. Or you might eat lunch at your desk every day, despite knowing that it is bad for your physical and mental health. Lace up your joggers instead and head outside for a short walk, which will improve not only your fitness but your mental clarity and concentration, too. These are just a few examples that can help improve your insulin resistance and PCOS symptoms.

To create a new habit, it can be useful to use mobile apps such as Productive or Momentum, keep a bullet journal, or use a simple Habit Tracker like the one on page 32. On average, it takes 66 days for a new habit to become automatic (Lally et al., 2010), meaning that you will not have to rely on apps or tricks to remember to follow them.

To use the Habit Tracker, jot down the habits you wish to focus on for the next week or month. This might mean fitting in a workout, avoiding sugar, or meditating for 15 minutes. Do not try to track too many habits at once—five or six is a manageable number for most people. For each day that you successfully complete your habit, mark it on the tracker. The more consecutive days you build up, the more likely you will stay on track, as you will not want to break your streak. Over time, your new habits will seamlessly become a permanent part of your lifestyle.

A WORD OF ENCOURAGEMENT

To practice self-compassion, say positive affirmations aloud. For example, "I must treat myself with kindness during this difficult journey," or "I am never alone."

YOUR HEALTHY HABIT TRACKER

MY NEW HEALTHY HABIT	M	Tu	W	Th	F	S	Su
	☐	☐	☐	☐	☐	☐	☐
	☐	☐	☐	☐	☐	☐	☐
	☐	☐	☐	☐	☐	☐	☐
	☐	☐	☐	☐	☐	☐	☐
	☐	☐	☐	☐	☐	☐	☐
	☐	☐	☐	☐	☐	☐	☐
	☐	☐	☐	☐	☐	☐	☐
	☐	☐	☐	☐	☐	☐	☐
	☐	☐	☐	☐	☐	☐	☐

30 Days of Intuitive Eating

It is important to realize that the goal is not to overcome insulin resistance within one month of beginning this diet. That approach would be unrealistic for most. Instead, your goal should be to discover a healthier way of eating with the help of the many nutritious recipes in this book, and also to implement new lifestyle and stress-relieving practices to improve your overall quality of life. These factors will let you overcome your insulin resistance over time, and in the short term, you can expect weight loss, higher energy, improved digestion, and a stronger body image.

Initially, as you learn to cement your new, healthy way of eating as a habit, it will be helpful to follow the four-week meal plan discussed in the following pages. At the end of the 30 days, you will understand the benefits of following such a diet, and may have already see improvements in some of your PCOS and insulin resistance symptoms, so you should feel motivated to continue.

At this time, the reasonable goal is to transition to a more intuitive style of eating. This means learning to eat according to your body's natural hunger and satiety signals, rather than following a specific plan. Here's how to eat intuitively:

Eat when you feel hungry, not when someone else (or the clock) tells you to. Continue to nourish your body with nutritious foods to maintain your positive progress.

Do not eat for emotional reasons. Many people turn to food during stressful times or even out of boredom. Whenever you think you are hungry, drink a glass of water and wait 15 minutes. During this time, partake in a non-food-related activity like going for a walk or calling a friend.

Practice mindfulness when you eat. This means shutting off the television, computer, or tablet while you eat, and instead focusing on the plate in front of you. Eat slowly and put your fork down after each bite.

Monitor how your body responds to certain foods. Pay attention to how you feel, physically and emotionally, after eating different types of foods. Although pizza and ice cream may make you feel great in the moment, they will likely make you feel sick and lethargic an hour or two later. Choose only foods that make you feel great.

Before you attempt intuitive eating, however, you must first learn healthy habits by following the four-week meal plan. Each of the following weekly meal plans is easy, convenient, and delicious. The ingredients are wholesome, easy-to-find, and affordable. The recipes are designed to be prepared quickly, and many of the recipes will generate leftovers. In fact, weekend meals will be cooked in bulk to allow you a day off from cooking midweek. The plans and recipes will provide all the tools you need to kick off your new, healthier life, free of insulin resistance and PCOS symptoms!

TARA'S TIPS FOR LOVING YOUR BODY– AND YOURSELF

When you initially receive your PCOS diagnosis, it is common to feel anger, frustration, and shame toward your body. Initially, I spoke very critically about myself and lost all sense of purpose, so I could no longer pursue my goals.

Thankfully, I learned how important it is to overcome this negative way of thinking. How you feel about your body directly affects your overall health; women with the poorest body image have the highest levels of cortisol from stress (Putterman and Linden, 2006). Treating yourself with love and kindness instead of anger and hostility will reduce your stress levels and help balance your hormone production. Knowing you are doing the right thing for your health will make it easier to maintain a healthy diet.

Here are my top 10 tips for cultivating greater love for your body:

Control what you can: Although it can be tempting to hide at home and wallow in self pity, remind yourself that PCOS can be controlled with a healthy diet and regular exercise. At times, my acne was so severe and painful that I cancelled social invitations out of embarrassment. But I discovered that by simply avoiding certain trigger foods and modifying my exercise regime, I could manage my acne, and I gained huge amounts of self-confidence in the process.

Accept that your body is unique: I accepted that my hormones were imbalanced, but I knew it was not permanent. Once my body was healthy again, my hormones would normalize and my menstrual cycle would return. I stopped comparing myself to others and was patient with my own healing process.

Practice self-compassion, expressing sympathy toward your own failures, inadequacies, and sufferings: Do not hold yourself to higher standards than you hold others to. Treat yourself with the same kindness, patience, and compassion you would extend to a loved one during a time of suffering.

Do not expect perfection: Love and respect yourself enough not only to stick to the principles of the diet, but also to forgive yourself during the times when you struggle. The road ahead may not be smooth sailing, but treating yourself with kindness will allow you to easily overcome the bumps along the way. Everyone fails; use it as an opportunity to learn and grow.

Allow nature to take its course: Instead of constantly obsessing over your hormone levels and PCOS symptoms, focus on how good it feels to follow a healthy diet and partake in a form of exercise you enjoy. In time, your hormones will respond, too, but not if you constantly berate your body for not responding fast enough.

Surround yourself with loving friends and family: The physical symptoms of PCOS—such as acne, weight gain, and excess body hair—can affect a woman's self-confidence. Spend time with loved ones who make you feel beautiful and who are also confident in their own skin and do not fixate on their appearance. Stop following social media accounts and any other media that make you feel bad about yourself.

Find a way to move that makes you feel good: Women with PCOS have a higher rate of anxiety and depression. This can be significantly reduced through regular exercise. Focus on what your body can do, instead of what it looks like.

Take five minutes each day to express gratitude: Give thanks for the good things in your life, whether that be access to water and healthy food, a loving partner and children, or a rewarding job.

Keep a journal: Use the journal to record your feelings each day and process any difficult moments in your journey. Jot down challenges and achievements.

Do not be ashamed to seek therapy: Almost everyone has psychological barriers that keep them from achieving full health and wellness; therapy can help you uncover and overcome them.

My favorite resources for building self-love and compassion are the Center for Young Women's Health and Self-Compassion websites. For more information about these sites and more, flip to the Resources section (see page 209).

THE 4-WEEK MEAL PLAN

The following four-week meal plan is designed to help you quickly get started on increasing the nutrient density of your diet and lowering your insulin resistance. The recipes can be found in chapters 3 through 10, and are designed to occasionally make use of leftovers to reduce the amount of cooking time you spend throughout the week. If you are just starting out with building your pantry ingredients, you may want to set a goal for the number of recipes you prepare each week. You can also look at each recipe to find the label designation ("Fertility Boost," "Lower Calorie," "Inflammation Fighter," etc.) and make replacements as needed. Most important, when you are using the meal plan, be flexible and feel free to make ingredient substitutions depending on what you have on hand.

YOUR FOUR-WEEK MEAL PLAN

1

	BREAKFAST	LUNCH	DINNER
Monday	Almond Flour Muffins (prepared Sunday)	Veggie Quinoa Mega Bowl	Meatless Monday: Cauliflower Fried Rice
Tuesday	Raspberry Hemp Breakfast Quinoa	Artichoke Millet Power Salad	Mushroom Barley Soup & Healthy and Easy Chicken Nuggets
Wednesday	Almond Flour Muffins	Mini Crustless Quiches	Leftover Cauliflower Fried Rice
Thursday	Coconut Cashew Green Smoothie	Veggie Quinoa Mega Bowl	Italian Baked Pork Chops with Fennel and Green Beans
Friday	Avocado Toast Five Ways	Artichoke Millet Power Salad	One-Pan Asparagus Eggs
Saturday	Pumpkin Pie Overnight Oats	Mini Crustless Quiches	Healthy and Easy Chicken Nuggets
Sunday	Quinoa Chia Pancakes	Mushroom Barley Soup & Almond Flour Muffins	Asian-Style Haddock in Parchment

YOUR FOUR-WEEK MEAL PLAN

2

	BREAKFAST	LUNCH	DINNER
Monday	Grain-Free Nut and Seed "Cereal" with Pears	Chickpea, Tomato, and Basil Salad	Meatless Monday: Kung Pao Tempeh
Tuesday	Slow Cooker Breakfast Casserole (prepared Sunday)	Leftover Kung Pao Tempeh	Almond Chicken and Greens Soup
Wednesday	Pumpkin Pie Overnight Oats	Leftover Almond Chicken and Greens Soup	Split Pea Falafel
Thursday	Slow Cooker Breakfast Casserole	Leftover Split Pea Falafel	Turkey Meatballs over Greens
Friday	Coconut Mango Smoothie	Chickpea, Tomato, and Basil Salad	Fish Tacos
Saturday	Blueberry Muffin Mug Cake	Asian Chicken Lettuce Wrap	Grilled Cauliflower Steaks with Mango and Black Bean Salsa
Sunday	Slow Cooker Breakfast Casserole	Asian Peanut Slaw	Mediterranean Shrimp Kabobs

YOUR FOUR-WEEK MEAL PLAN

3

	BREAKFAST	LUNCH	DINNER
Monday	Pumpkin Pie Overnight Oats	Mini Crustless Quiches (prepared Saturday)	Meatless Monday: Tofu Kale Scramble
Tuesday	Slow Cooker Breakfast Casserole (prepared Sunday)	Chickpea, Tomato, and Basil Salad	Chicken and Pepper Fajitas
Wednesday	Avocado Toast Five Ways	Moroccan Spiced Buckwheat Salad	Black Bean and Chickpea Veggie Chili
Thursday	Slow Cooker Breakfast Casserole (prepared Sunday)	Chickpea, Tomato, and Basil Salad	Cod with Sugar Snap Peas
Friday	Raspberry Hemp Breakfast Quinoa	Mason Jar Taco Salad	Baked Broccoli and Bean Burgers
Saturday	Quinoa Chia Pancakes	Mini Crustless Quiches	Open-Face Turkey Veggie Burgers
Sunday	Slow Cooker Breakfast Casserole	Persian Cucumber Salad	Grilled Salmon with Pomegranate, Mint, and Pine Nut Couscous

YOUR FOUR-WEEK MEAL PLAN

4	BREAKFAST	LUNCH	DINNER
Monday	Raspberry Hemp Breakfast Quinoa	Artichoke Millet Power Salad	Meatless Monday: Spinach, Sweet Potato, and Lentil Dal
Tuesday	Blueberry Muffin Mug Cake	Leftover Spinach, Sweet Potato, and Lentil Dal	Rosemary and Almond–Crusted Baked Chicken
Wednesday	Raspberry Hemp Breakfast Quinoa	Mason Jar Taco Salad	Halibut with Lentils and Mustard Sauce
Thursday	Pumpkin Pie Overnight Oats	Artichoke Millet Power Salad	Stir-Fried Pork and Vegetables
Friday	Peaches and Greens Smoothie	Mason Jar Taco Salad	Miso Tofu Soup & Healthy and Easy Chicken Nuggets
Saturday	Quinoa Chia Pancakes	Salmon, Apple, and Avocado Wrap	Navy Bean and Quinoa Loaf
Sunday	Slow Cooker Breakfast Casserole	Leftover Navy Bean and Quinoa Loaf	Tilapia and Vegetable Packets

Pantry Staples

Keeping a well-stocked, real-food kitchen is essential to a healthy lifestyle. Have nutritious foods at your fingertips at all times, and no processed foods to fall back on.

The following foods are key staple ingredients you will need for preparing the recipes in this book. Fill your pantry with these basics, and then shop for the more perishable items once or twice a week. Having a fully stocked, real-food pantry can take time, so plan what you will buy first, based on the recipes you decide to prepare. Look for sales, buy in bulk, and choose organic and grass-fed or pasture-raised whenever possible. When making budgeting decisions about your produce purchases, use the Environmental Working Group's Dirty Dozen and Clean Fifteen lists, which rank fruits and vegetables by their pesticide load in a given year (see Appendix C, page 207).

Grains: Millet, brown rice, quinoa, old-fashioned rolled oats, buckwheat, sprouted bread, and sprouted tortillas

Beans and legumes: Dried lentils and canned beans (black beans, chickpeas, white/cannellini beans, butter/lima beans, and black-eyed peas)

Flours and baking: Coconut flour, almond flour, chickpea flour, panko bread crumbs, baking powder, and baking soda

Oils and vinegars: Olive oil, coconut oil, white wine vinegar, cider vinegar, and balsamic vinegar

Nuts and seeds: Flaxseed meal (ground flaxseed), chia seeds, sliced almonds, pumpkin seeds, hemp seeds, natural peanut butter, and natural almond butter

Seasonings and sweeteners: Stevia, unsweetened cocoa powder, vanilla extract, Bragg's liquid aminos, Sriracha sauce, miso, and a gluten-free, soy-based all-purpose seasoning sauce

Herbs and spices: Basil, dill, oregano, rosemary, chives, garlic, sage, parsley, cinnamon, nutmeg, ginger, black pepper, cloves, and turmeric

Refrigerator: Plain unsweetened nonfat Greek yogurt, eggs, tempeh, tofu, unsweetened vanilla almond milk, lean organic meats (pork, chicken, and turkey)

Freezer: Frozen blueberries, raspberries, kale, spinach, riced cauliflower, edamame, and green peas

Seafood: Haddock, shrimp, salmon, and halibut

Shelf-stable: Unsweetened applesauce and pure canned pumpkin

Fresh fruits: Pears, apples, berries, and avocados

Fresh vegetables: Tomatoes, mushrooms, bell peppers, onion, zucchini, carrots, cucumbers, baby salad greens, snap peas, edamame, celery, cauliflower (whole and riced), Brussels sprouts, portobello mushrooms, broccoli, acorn squash, green beans, and cabbage

Teas: Chai and green

SHOPPING GUIDE

Eating home-cooked meals made with fresh food just can't be beat when you want to improve your health, know what's really in your food, and have more control over your portion size. The challenge with this for many people, however, is that grocery shopping seems like an expensive and time-consuming chore. Although it may be tempting to choose cheaper, processed foods to save money, there are many ways to eat healthy, organic, whole foods on a budget. Here are 5 tips to get you started:

Plan your meals and shop wisely: Planning your meals is a surefire way to improve the quality of your diet. Set aside time each week to plan out what you will eat every day, including snacks. Using your plan, do a pantry inventory and prepare a shopping list so that you have the items you need on hand. Planning saves you money by cutting down on food waste and eliminates the stress of "What's for dinner?" At the grocery store, stick to your list and shop the perimeter of the store first, since that is where the whole foods are generally located. Avoid shopping when you are hungry, because it can lead to unintended, expensive purchases.

Shop locally and seasonally: Local, in-season produce is generally cheaper, more nutritious, and more flavorful than out-of-season produce and fruits and vegetables that have traveled long distances to get to your grocery store. Shop your local farmers' markets or join a community-supported agriculture (CSA) program. By joining a CSA, you will have access to fresh, locally grown foods, although your choices may be more limited to what's in season. If you want to join a CSA, go to localharvest.org, click on "CSA," and type in your zip code to receive contact information for the farm closest to you.

Be freezer-friendly: Quick-frozen fruits and vegetables are picked and packaged at the peak of freshness. Just as nutritious as fresh, frozen produce is available year round and often is sold in large bags. With frozen produce you gain the advantage of being able to take out only what you are going to use and keep the rest for later, without spoiling. Reducing produce waste is a great way to save money.

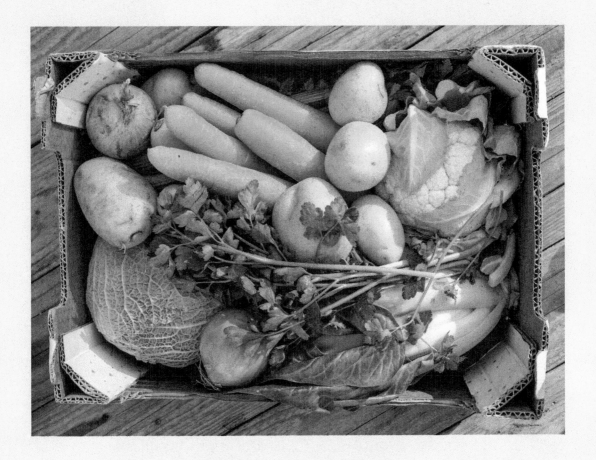

Prepare meatless meals more often:
Start a new family tradition by having "Meatless Mondays," when you serve vegetarian meals. Plant proteins like legumes, beans, and soy are inexpensive yet nutritious and easy to prepare. Replacing meat once or twice a week with plant protein can reduce your grocery bill.

Buy in bulk: Buying some foods in bulk quantities can save you a lot of money. Grains (such as brown rice, millet, barley, and oats), nuts and seeds, and dried legumes and beans are all available in bulk. They also keep for a long time when stored in a dark, cool place in airtight containers. These are all staple foods that are relatively inexpensive and can be used in a variety of healthy meals.

Essential Equipment

Cooking is easier and faster when you have the right equipment on hand. If your kitchen is stocked with the basics, you can probably prepare most of the recipes in this book. But there are a few special tools you may want to purchase, which will help save you time, allow you to cook in bulk, and expand your culinary horizons. You don't have to buy all of these items at once and can accumulate kitchen equipment over time. Building up a set of tools that feels comfortable for you can take time and depends on your preferences and budget. The following is a list of essential kitchen tools and equipment for you to consider:

Good-quality knives: If you have never worked with a good-quality knife, it may be a game changer for you. Whether you are dealing with fruit, vegetables, herbs, or meat, you are going to need to chop, slice, or dice at some point. The two most import-ant knives in your arsenal are a good-quality chef's knife to tackle the big stuff and a par-ing knife that can handle the little things.

Cutting board: A wooden cutting board will be easy on your blades, keeping your knives in top condition. Dedicated cutting boards—one for meat only, seafood, and poultry, and one for produce only—are ideal, but not necessarily practical when funds are tight. Just be sure to sanitize your board after working with raw meats or seafood to avoid cross-contamination.

Mixing bowls: You might be surprised by how much mixing you will do, so look for durable nesting bowls that can handle large and small volumes. If possible, choose ones with lids, which make them perfect for keeping leftovers.

Measuring cups and spoons: You'll need different measuring cups to measure dry and liquid ingredients, because mea-surements for each are designed slightly differently to accommodate the qualities of dry and liquid ingredients. Wet measures have a spout for easy pouring; look for tempered glass. Dry-ingredient measuring cups are designed to be filled to the top and leveled off; look for stainless steel. You will also need a set of measuring spoons.

Baking sheets: Look for baking sheets that have a 1-inch rim, designed to catch juices from roasting vegetables, meat, fish, poultry, and pizza. Cookie sheets are for baking cookies; they are flat with a rim that you can grab at one end. Baking sheets commonly come in metal, ceramic, and silicone.

Baking dishes: Baking dishes make roast chickens, casseroles, and desserts all possible. They are even useful for serving straight from the oven to the table. Baking dishes come in glass, metal, ceramic, and enamel-coated cast iron, and those with lids are great for storing leftovers. Try to have a variety of sizes on hand.

Pots and pans: A nonstick saucepan makes cleanup a breeze and requires less oil to keep food from sticking or burning. The recipes in this book require saucepans in a variety of sizes to accommodate sauces, soups, and stews. To get started, choose three sizes: 2-, 4-, and 8-quart saucepans or pots with lids. Quality really counts, so choose sturdy pots; thin, cheap metals will warp, dent, and may burn both you and your food. Nontoxic, eco-friendly options include glass, ceramic, stainless steel, and Green nonstick cookware.

Nonstick skillet/frying pan: A good nonstick skillet is indispensable. You can brown, fry, and sauté with one. A large one (9 to 10 inches) will be used for most of the recipes and is the perfect size if you are feeding a small family.

Slow cooker: A slow cooker or crockpot has many advantages and is a great way to save time while preparing a nutritious meal. Compared with a standard oven, this appliance uses only a small amount of electricity, and because it cooks food using low heat over a long time period, it actually retains more of the nutrients in your food. Slow cookers can be used for breakfast casseroles, steel-cut oats, soups, stews, roasts, and even desserts.

Food processor: A food processor is another essential time-saving device and can make chopping, slicing, grating, and dicing a breeze. Tips will be provided for using it to purée soups, grind oats into flour, and make your own nut butter. Some recipes in this book that are easily and quickly prepared using a food processor are hummus and pesto.

High-speed blender: A high-speed blender, depending on the model, can be used in place of a food processor for basic tasks like puréeing and dicing. A good blender makes all the difference when preparing whole-food smoothies and handling ingredients like nuts and fresh fruits and vegetables. It's also a great tool for processing soups into velvety purées.

Other tools: Other items you should have on hand are an instant-read meat thermometer, timer, colander, wooden spoons, slotted spoon, ladle, spatula, whisk, can opener, vegetable peeler, grater, oven mitts, pot holders, kitchen towels, and apron.

Troubleshooting Tips

Since PCOS cannot yet be completely cured, it is important to maintain your new healthy habits for life so that your symptoms don't return. Following are 10 common problems you may encounter once you begin the Insulin Resistance Diet for PCOS, and tips for overcoming them:

Lack of time: All of the recipes require less than 15 minutes of preparation, and many meals can be cooked in bulk amounts (especially on the weekend, when you have more time). Freeze some of your leftovers so you always have food on standby when you are too tired to cook. Also, try buying pre-prepared ingredients (such as chopped fresh vegetables). Once you have finished the four-week meal plan, set aside 10 minutes per week to plan out all of your meals for the week ahead.

Inability to cook: The recipes in this book are extremely simple for every cook—even someone who has never used an oven before. Cooking can be a fun activity, once you learn a few basic recipes.

Cravings for processed foods: Remember that, over time, your cravings will lessen. Keep nutritious snacks in your fridge and pantry for those moments when cravings strike, and remind yourself that a fleeting craving is not worth undoing all your hard work.

Dislike of healthy foods: You can retrain your taste buds to appreciate fresh fruits and vegetables, healthy grains, and lean proteins. Experiment with seasonings and lots of different healthy recipes. Your new diet should be flavorful and exciting. Sometimes you may have to give yourself a little tough love, and remind yourself that you should be eating for optimal health.

Eating in restaurants: Almost every restaurant offers a healthy option, even if you have to order off the menu. Ask for grilled meat or fish with basic seasoning, served alongside fresh vegetables with dressing on the side. Avoid those restaurants and cafés that will be too tempting for you.

Dislike of water: Plain water can be boring if you drink it all the time. Try infusing your water with cucumber, ginger, lemon, lime, mint, or orange. Make iced coolers. Green and herbal teas are also great options.

Unsupportive family members and friends: If your loved ones try to lead you astray with processed foods, remind them that you are following this diet to improve your health, and that indulging in high-sugar and high-fat foods goes directly against that.

Expense of healthy eating: Many people mistakenly assume that it is expensive to eat healthy. While it is true that organic meats and fresh fruits and vegetables can be expensive, your grocery bill should be balanced out by the reduction in processed foods—not to mention fewer medical bills down the line! Buying in bulk, following a meal plan, and shopping at local farmers' markets will also help you stick to a budget.

Off-plan meals: You cannot be expected to perfectly conform to the diet outlined in this book for the rest of your life. Occasional slip-ups will happen, and there will be times where you can intuitively choose to go off the plan. The trick is to make sure these occasions happen infrequently, and not allow one off-plan meal to turn into multiple days off the plan. No one except you will know if you slip up, so you must hold yourself accountable and remember why this diet is critical for your health and happiness.

Overcoming an emotional relationship with food: For some people, it is not simple to switch to a healthy lifestyle, even when they are aware of the health benefits. Some people have deep emotional connections with food, and it is something they turn to in times of stress or boredom. If you are one of these people, it is important to focus on rebuilding your psychological health by finding non-food-related activities that give you pleasure, and also to consider therapy if your food issues border on disordered eating behaviors. Do not attempt to change too many factors at once, and always treat your body with kindness and forgiveness.

II The Recipes

"Let food be thy medicine and medicine be thy food."

–Hippocrates

Each of the recipes in this book is designed to be nutrient dense and include ingredients that are familiar yet rich in essential vitamins, minerals, fiber, and phytochemicals.

Each recipe has one of the following labels at the top:

FERTILITY BOOST This signifies that the ingredients used in the recipe can support fertility as well as a healthy pregnancy.

LOWER CALORIE Weight management in the midst of hormonal disturbances can be challenging. Look for this label, which indicates that the recipe is beneficial for weight loss and/or includes nutrients that can boost metabolism or satiety.

INFLAMMATION FIGHTER Whole, unprocessed foods are rich in inflammation-fighting nutrients. When you see this label, it means that the recipe's ingredients help fight inflammation in the body.

DAIRY FREE This recipe designation signifies that no milk products are used.

GLUTEN FREE This label means that none of the ingredients used in the recipe contain gluten.

Each recipe also contains a tip at the bottom:

FERTILITY BOOST TIP This tip provides additional information for women trying to conceive, regarding substitutions or additions that can be made to increase the content of nutrients specifically shown to be important for fertility.

INFLAMMATION FIGHTER TIP This kind of tip discusses ways to increase the anti-inflammatory effects of the recipe through the use of additional ingredients or substitutions.

LOWER CALORIE TIP This tip offers suggestions on how to reduce the overall calorie content and/or increase the protein content of the recipe.

INGREDIENT TIP Some recipes include a tip with information on how to select, work with, or prepare certain ingredients.

COOKING TIP This tip contains shortcuts for reducing cooking time or additional information that will make the dish easier to prepare.

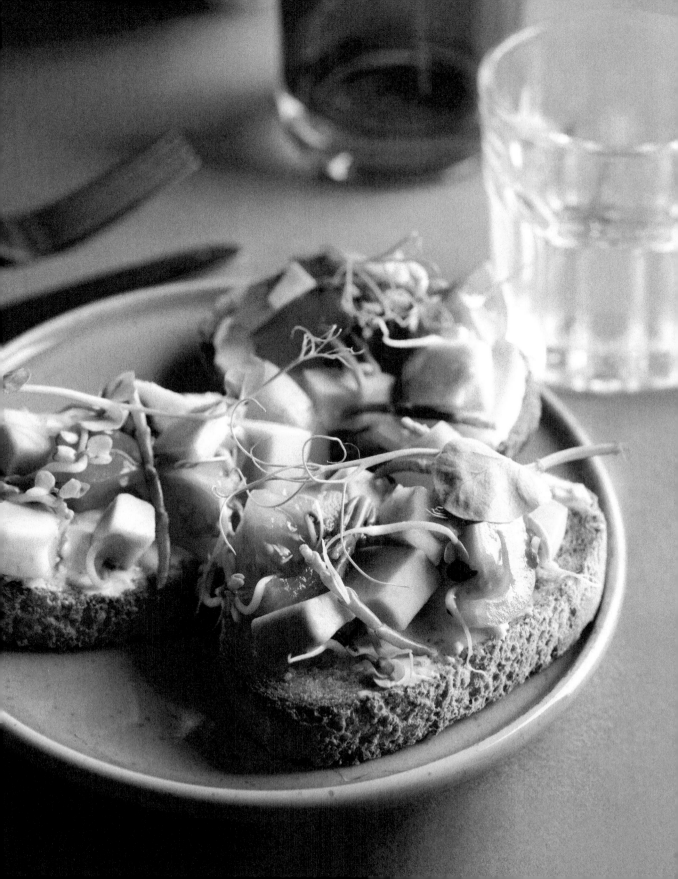

3

Breakfast

Coconut Cashew Green Smoothie

DAIRY FREE, GLUTEN FREE

1 (13.5-ounce) can light
    coconut milk
1 medium apple, cored
    and chopped
1-inch piece fresh ginger,
    peeled and minced
1 teaspoon ground cinnamon
1 teaspoon vanilla extract
⅓ cup frozen green peas
1 cup stemmed and
    chopped kale
1 cup baby spinach leaves
½ cup dry-roasted cashews
½ cup ice cubes

SERVES 2 | PREP TIME: 5 MINUTES

Cashews and peas are both low in glycemic load and high in protein. The kale and spinach give you a couple of servings of veggies for the day, and the apple adds heart-healthy fiber and beneficial phytochemicals. The coconut milk is a healthy fat that will help keep you feeling satisfied, and the cinnamon is a natural blood-sugar stabilizer.

1. In a blender, combine the coconut milk, apple, ginger, cinnamon, vanilla, peas, kale, spinach, cashews, and ice.

2. Blend on high until smooth.

3. Immediately pour the mixture into 2 tall glasses and serve.

LOWER CALORIE TIP: *For a higher protein, lower calorie smoothie, replace the coconut milk with unsweetened almond milk and add 6 ounces of plain unsweetened Greek yogurt. Frozen peas are used to provide unprocessed plant protein, but instead, you could add a serving of your favorite protein powder.*

PER SERVING: CALORIES: 668; CARBS: 38G; GLYCEMIC LOAD: 13; FIBER: 6G; SODIUM: 80MG; PROTEIN: 13G; FAT: 57G; SATURATED FAT: 39G

Cherry Smoothie Bowl

FERTILITY BOOST, INFLAMMATION FIGHTER, GLUTEN FREE

2 cups frozen cherries

½ cup old-fashioned rolled oats, soaked in ½ cup unsweetened almond milk overnight

1 cup plain nonfat Greek yogurt

1 tablespoon chia seeds

1 teaspoon vanilla extract

1 tablespoon natural almond butter

2 teaspoons hemp seeds

½ cup fresh berries

2 teaspoons sliced almonds

SERVES 2 | PREP TIME: 5 MINUTES

Smoothie bowls are another great high-protein breakfast to start your day. They can be made with a variety of ingredients to provide an assortment of flavors and tastes. The main difference between a smoothie and a smoothie bowl is that smoothie bowls are thicker, meant to be eaten in a bowl with a spoon, and generally contain a number of toppings. This recipe features cherries, a low-GI fruit that is high in beta carotene, vitamin C, potassium, folate, iron, magnesium, and fiber. The combination of cherries, oats, and Greek yogurt creates a thick, creamy, satisfying, and nutritious way to start your day.

1. In a blender, combine the cherries, soaked oats, yogurt, chia seeds, vanilla, and almond butter. Blend until smooth. Pour into 2 bowls.

2. Top each bowl with 1 teaspoon hemp seeds, ¼ cup fresh berries, and 1 teaspoon sliced almonds. Serve.

INFLAMMATION FIGHTER TIP: *One of the biggest benefits of cherries comes from powerful antioxidants known as anthocyanins, which have the ability to reduce inflammation and the risk factors for diabetes. To reap the benefits, aim to have one serving of cherries each day. Sample serving sizes are ½ cup unsweetened dried, 1 cup fresh, 1 cup frozen, 1 cup 100-percent pure unsweetened cherry juice.*

PER SERVING: CALORIES: 488; CARBS: 62G; GLYCEMIC LOAD: 26; FIBER: 11G; SODIUM: 128MG; PROTEIN: 18G; FAT: 18G; SATURATED FAT: 3G

Avocado Toast Five Ways

FERTILITY BOOST, INFLAMMATION FIGHTER

5 slices sprouted whole
grain bread
3 medium avocados, pitted
and cubed

OPTIONAL TOPPINGS:
1 hard-boiled egg, sliced
Salt
Freshly ground black pepper
¼ cup unsweetened plain
Greek yogurt, divided
3 strawberries, hulled
and sliced
¼ cup canned chickpeas
(garbanzo beans), drained
and rinsed
1 teaspoon Sriracha sauce
¼ yellow bell pepper, sliced
¼ cup canned black beans,
drained and rinsed
2 tablespoons fresh
cilantro leaves
1 medium tomato, chopped
Handful sprouts and
micro greens

MAKES 5 SLICES | PREP TIME: 10 MINUTES

Avocados provide nearly 20 essential nutrients, including fiber, potassium, vitamin E, B vitamins, and folic acid, a B vitamin essential for preventing neural tube defects. Rich in carotenoids, phytosterols, and omega-3 fatty acids, their unique nutritional profile offers powerful anti-inflammatory benefits. Research (Wien et al., 2013) has also shown that eating half an avocado with meals leads to long-term satiety, or a greater feeling of fullness, which can help with weight loss by suppressing appetite. Presented five ways, this recipe is sure to please even the pickiest eater.

1. Toast the bread slices.

2. In a medium bowl, mash the avocados with a fork. (Or leave the avocado in cubes, if you like.)

3. Spread or scatter the avocado on the 5 slices of toasted bread, dividing it evenly.

4. Top each of the 5 avocado toasts in one of the following ways:

Avocado, Egg, Salt, Freshly Ground Black Pepper: Place the sliced egg on top of the avocado. Season with salt and pepper.

Avocado, Greek Yogurt, Strawberries: Spread or dollop 2 tablespoons of the Greek yogurt on top of the avocado. Top with the sliced strawberries.

Avocado, Chickpeas, Sriracha Sauce: Layer the chickpeas on top of the avocado. Top with a drizzle of Sriracha sauce.

Avocado, Yellow Bell Pepper, Black Beans, Cilantro: Layer the sliced bell pepper slices on the avocado mash. Between each pepper slice, add a row of black beans. Sprinkle with the cilantro leaves.

Avocado, Greek Yogurt, Tomato, and Microgreens: Spread or dollop the remaining 2 tablespoons of Greek yogurt on top of the avocado. Top with the chopped tomato and microgreens. Season with salt and freshly ground black pepper.

INFLAMMATION FIGHTER TIP: *When choosing bread, look for a loaf that contains primarily sprouted grains and legumes. In their sprouting form, grains and legumes have an enhanced nutritional value, because sprouting boosts the protein, fiber, folate, vitamin C, vitamin E, and beta-carotene content. Sprouting also reduces the amount of harmful substances that inhibit nutrient absorption and makes grains easier to digest.*

PER SERVING: (Avocado, Egg, Salt, Freshly Ground Black Pepper) CALORIES: 205; CARBS: 19G; GLYCEMIC LOAD: 7; FIBER: 7G; SODIUM: 158MG; PROTEIN: 5G; FAT: 14G; SATURATED FAT: 2G

(Avocado, Greek Yogurt, Strawberries) CALORIES: 236; CARBS: 24G; GLYCEMIC LOAD: 9; FIBER: 8G; SODIUM: 132MG; PROTEIN: 7G; FAT: 15G; SATURATED FAT: 2G

(Avocado, Chickpeas, Sriracha Sauce) CALORIES: 272; CARBS: 30G; GLYCEMIC LOAD: 11; FIBER: 10G; SODIUM: 245MG; PROTEIN: 9G; FAT: 15G; SATURATED FAT: 2G

(Avocado, Yellow Bell Pepper, Black Beans, Cilantro) CALORIES: 275; CARBS: 32G; GLYCEMIC LOAD: 11; FIBER: 11G; SODIUM: 132MG; PROTEIN: 9G; FAT: 14G; SATURATED FAT: 2G

(Avocado, Greek Yogurt, Tomato, and Microgreens) CALORIES: 250; CARBS: 27G; GLYCEMIC LOAD: 10; FIBER: 9G; SODIUM: 131MG; PROTEIN: 8G; FAT: 15G; SATURATED FAT: 2G

Raspberry Hemp Breakfast Quinoa

INFLAMMATION FIGHTER, DAIRY FREE, GLUTEN FREE

1 cup uncooked quinoa,
    rinsed (see Ingredient Tip)
2 cups unsweetened
    almond milk
1 teaspoon vanilla extract
1 teaspoon ground cinnamon
1 tablespoon natural
    almond butter
4 tablespoons hemp seeds
2 cups fresh or frozen and
    thawed raspberries

SERVES 4 | PREP TIME: 5 MINUTES | COOK TIME: 20 MINUTES

For a new go-to hot cereal, try quinoa for breakfast. This inflammation-fighting, high-protein, grain-like seed provides a satisfying meal in the morning. Hemp seeds and almond butter provide plant protein, fiber, and healthy unsaturated fats to keep blood sugar steady. The combination of cinnamon, vanilla, and high-fiber raspberries make this a creamy, sweet dish that will fuel you for hours.

1. Put the quinoa in a medium saucepan over medium heat. Toast for 2 minutes, stirring constantly.

2. Stir in the almond milk, vanilla, and cinnamon. Increase the heat to medium high and bring the mixture to a slow boil, stirring constantly. Reduce the heat to low and cover the pan. Cook for 15 minutes or until the quinoa has absorbed the liquid.

3. Remove the pan from the heat and fluff with a fork.

4. While the quinoa is still warm, stir in the almond butter and hemp seeds. Gently fold in the raspberries.

5. Serve warm.

INGREDIENT TIP: *To prep the quinoa, put it in a fine-mesh sieve and rinse it well under cool running water. Rub the quinoa between your hands for 1 minute to wash off the natural bitter coating. Drain.*

COOKING TIP: *For a make-ahead breakfast, prepare this quinoa dish (omitting the raspberries) and store it covered in the refrigerator for up to 4 days. When ready to eat, heat the quinoa mixture and top it with the raspberries.*

PER SERVING: CALORIES: 424; CARBS: 66G; GLYCEMIC LOAD: 28; FIBER: 9G; SODIUM: 74MG; PROTEIN: 13G; FAT: 12G; SATURATED FAT: 1G

Slow Cooker Breakfast Casserole

FERTILITY BOOST, LOWER CALORIE, GLUTEN FREE

Olive oil cooking spray
8 eggs
½ cup unsweetened
    almond milk
1 garlic clove, minced
¼ teaspoon salt
¼ teaspoon freshly ground
    black pepper
2 cups riced cauliflower
    (see Cooking Tip;
    from ½ head)
1 cup thawed frozen spinach
1 small yellow onion, diced
1 cup nutritional yeast
Chopped tomatoes,
    for garnish
Chopped fresh flat-leaf
    parsley, for garnish

COOKING TIP: *Riced cauliflower is a popular low-carb grain replacement. In this recipe, it takes the place of high-glycemic-index hash browns. Riced cauliflower is easy to make by pulsing the florets in a food processor (or blender). To save time, you can find riced cauliflower in the produce and frozen sections of most supermarkets.*

SERVES 4 | PREP TIME: 10 MINUTES| COOK TIME: 5 TO 7 HOURS ON LOW, 1½ TO 2 HOURS ON HIGH

This fertility-boosting recipe is loaded with choline, which can reduce harmful gene effects that may result in birth defects. Most women don't get enough choline. Many prenatal vitamins don't even include choline. Egg yolks and cauliflower are rich in choline. In this casserole, nutritional yeast takes the place of high-fat dairy cheese, boosting the B-vitamin content even further.

1. Spray a 6-quart slow cooker insert with olive oil cooking spray.

2. In a medium bowl, lightly beat together the eggs, almond milk, garlic, salt, and pepper.

3. Place about one-third of the cauliflower in an even layer on the bottom of the slow cooker, and top it with about one-third of the spinach, onion, and nutritional yeast. Repeat the layers two more times. Pour the egg mixture over the contents.

4. Cook on low for 5 to 7 hours or on high for 1½ to 2 hours, until the eggs are set and the top is browned.

5. Turn off the slow cooker.

6. Cut the casserole into 4 wedges and transfer them to serving plates.

7. Garnish with chopped tomatoes and fresh parsley.

8. Serve warm.

PER SERVING: CALORIES: 218; CARBS: 12G; GLYCEMIC LOAD: 4; FIBER: 7G; SODIUM: 326MG; PROTEIN: 22G; FAT: 10G; SATURATED FAT: 3G

Grain-Free Nut and Seed "Cereal" with Pears

INFLAMMATION FIGHTER, GLUTEN FREE

2 tablespoons sliced almonds

2 tablespoons hemp seeds

2 tablespoons almond meal

2 tablespoons flaxseed meal

½ teaspoon ground cinnamon

½ teaspoon vanilla extract

1 cup plain nonfat
   Greek yogurt

1 large pear, sliced

SERVES 2 | PREP TIME: 5 MINUTES

This hearty, quick and easy, grain-free cereal gives you plenty of inflammation-fighting omega-3s and high-quality protein for long lasting energy. The low-glycemic-load pear gives you heart-healthy soluble fiber and a serving of fruit, and the cinnamon acts to stabilize blood sugar.

1. In a medium bowl, combine the almonds, hemp seeds, almond meal, flaxseed meal, cinnamon, and vanilla.

2. Divide the mixture between two cereal bowls. Top each with one-half of the yogurt and one-half of the pear slices.

3. Serve immediately.

INFLAMMATION FIGHTER TIP: *Nuts and seeds are rich in healthy unsaturated fats, including the essential omega-3 fatty acids that act as powerful anti-inflammatories in the body. To give this recipe even more inflammation-fighting power, add 2 tablespoons of chia seeds, increase the cinnamon to 1 teaspoon, and add grated fresh ginger.*

PER SERVING: CALORIES: 366; CARBS: 27G; GLYCEMIC LOAD: 8; FIBER: 7G; SODIUM: 95MG; PROTEIN: 18G; FAT: 21G; SATURATED FAT: 2G

Quinoa Chia Pancakes

INFLAMMATION FIGHTER, GLUTEN FREE

3 cups cooked quinoa
2 tablespoons coconut flour
1 cup unsweetened
  almond milk
1 teaspoon vanilla extract
4 eggs
2 tablespoons chia seeds
1 tablespoon baking powder
1 teaspoon ground ginger
Pinch salt
Olive oil cooking spray
1 cup fresh raspberries or
  other berries, (optional)

SERVES 4 | PREP TIME: 10 MINUTES | COOK TIME: 15 MINUTES

Traditional pancakes are a carbohydrate bomb and can send your blood sugar into a tailspin. If you've been missing a golden stack on lazy mornings, try this low-glycemic recipe. This recipe is high in complete protein from quinoa, rich in anti-inflammatory omega-3 fatty acids from chia seeds, and has the added benefit of ginger, a spice known to support healthy blood sugar and metabolism.

1. In a blender, combine the quinoa, coconut flour, almond milk, vanilla, and eggs. Blend on high speed until a smooth batter forms.

2. Add the chia seeds, baking powder, ginger, and salt. Pulse a few times to combine the ingredients. The batter will be thick.

3. Coat a large skillet with olive oil cooking spray and place it over medium heat.

4. Pour about ¼ cup of batter into the skillet for each pancake, and cook for about 4 minutes, until the edges are firm and the bottoms are golden. Flip the pancakes and cook for about 3 minutes, until the second side is golden and the pancakes are cooked through. Remove to a warm plate. Repeat with the remaining batter.

5. Serve warm, topped with raspberries (if using).

LOWER CALORIE TIP: *To lower the calorie count of this recipe while keeping the protein high, replace the 4 eggs with ¾ cup fresh egg whites. These pancakes also make a great portable post-workout snack, because of their balance of high-quality protein, healthy carbs, and fiber—much healthier than packaged protein bars.*

PER SERVING: CALORIES: 342; CARBS: 44G; GLYCEMIC LOAD: 17; FIBER: 9G; SODIUM: 395MG; PROTEIN: 14G; FAT: 13G; SATURATED FAT: 2G

Blueberry Muffin Mug Cake

LOWER CALORIE, INFLAMMATION FIGHTER

2 tablespoons oat flour
1 tablespoon coconut flour
1 tablespoon almond flour
½ teaspoon baking powder
½ teaspoon ground nutmeg
1 large egg, lightly beaten
½ teaspoon vanilla extract
1 tablespoon unsweetened
    applesauce or
    pumpkin purée
2 tablespoons unsweetened
    almond milk
2 tablespoons frozen
    blueberries
Olive oil cooking spray

SERVES 1 | PREP TIME: 5 MINUTES | COOK TIME: 1 TO 2 MINUTES

The magic of mug cakes is in the small ingredient proportions you need. The small size and cook time mean that they are perfect for experimentation and a quick breakfast, snack, or dessert. This quick and easy recipe is low in calories yet high in blood sugar–stabilizing nutrients and protein from the egg and the nutmeg. Blueberries add beneficial phytochemicals that can help reduce inflammation.

1. In a large bowl, stir together the oat flour, coconut flour, almond flour, baking powder, and nutmeg.

2. Add the egg, vanilla, applesauce, and almond milk to the flour mixture, and stir until smooth. Gently fold in the blueberries.

3. Coat the sides of a large mug (12 ounces or larger) with olive oil cooking spray. Spoon the batter into the mug.

4. Microwave on high for 50 seconds, then stop and check to see if the batter is set. Continue to microwave, 10 seconds at a time, until the batter is set, about 2 minutes total, depending on the microwave strength.

5. Once the cake is set, let it cool slightly, then transfer it to a plate.

6. Serve warm.

FERTILITY BOOST TIP: *Replace the almond flour with flaxseed meal for additional omega-3 fatty acids and lignin (a type of phytochemical). Omega-3 fats benefit the development of a baby's brain and nervous system and help reduce the risk of premature birth.*

PER SERVING: CALORIES: 308; CARBS: 29G; GLYCEMIC LOAD: 16; FIBER: 1G; SODIUM: 249MG; PROTEIN: 10G; FAT: 18G; SATURATED FAT: 3G

Pumpkin Pie Overnight Oats

LOWER CALORIE, GLUTEN FREE

½ cup nonfat plain
   Greek yogurt
¼ cup unsweetened
   pumpkin purée
2 tablespoons unsweetened
   almond milk
¼ cup old-fashioned
   rolled oats
1 tablespoon chia seeds
½ teaspoon vanilla extract
¼ teaspoon ground cinnamon
⅛ teaspoon ground nutmeg
⅛ teaspoon ground ginger
Granulated stevia
1 tablespoon sliced almonds

SERVES 1 | PREP TIME: 5 MINUTES, PLUS 4 HOURS OR MORE
TO CHILL

Oats are one of the healthiest grains you can eat. They are a gluten-free whole grain and a great source of important vitamins, minerals, fiber, and antioxidants. Because oatmeal has a low glycemic index, it can help maintain steady blood sugar levels. Eating oatmeal promotes heart health by helping keep bad cholesterol in check. This super-easy recipe tastes like a slice of pumpkin pie straight from the Thanksgiving table and can easily be doubled or tripled.

1. In a medium bowl or 8-ounce mason jar, combine the yogurt, pumpkin, almond milk, oats, chia seeds, vanilla, cinnamon, nutmeg, ginger, and stevia. Mix thoroughly.

2. Cover and refrigerate for at least 4 hours, or until the oats are soft.

3. Top with the almonds.

FERTILITY BOOST TIP: *To give this recipe a fertility boost, stir in 1 tablespoon of wheat germ. This nutritional powerhouse is high in protein and fiber, and is an excellent source of folate, a B vitamin critical for preventing birth defects, and zinc, which is necessary for proper growth and development.*

PER SERVING: CALORIES: 397; CARBS: 48G; GLYCEMIC LOAD: 21;
FIBER: 13G; SODIUM: 95MG; PROTEIN: 18G; FAT: 14G; SATURATED FAT: 3G

Almond Flour Muffins

INFLAMMATION FIGHTER, DAIRY FREE, GLUTEN FREE

2½ cups almond flour
   or almond meal
1 teaspoon baking soda
½ teaspoon salt
3 eggs
⅓ cup unsweetened
   applesauce or
   pumpkin purée
2 tablespoons agave nectar
2 tablespoons
   coconut oil, melted
1 teaspoon white vinegar
1 teaspoon vanilla extract
1 cup chopped fresh fruit
   (optional)

MAKES 12 | PREP TIME: 5 MINUTES
COOK TIME: 15 TO 20 MINUTES

These gluten-free, inflammation-fighting muffins not only taste terrific, but can also provide you with a number of health benefits. Almonds are high in magnesium, a mineral that can improve insulin resistance, and several studies (e.g., Mori et al., 2011) have shown that incorporating almonds into the diet can lessen the rise in blood sugar after meals, reduce levels of hemoglobin A1C, support healthy cholesterol levels, and help with weight management. Eating almonds along with a high-glycemic-index food can also lessen the rise in blood sugar after eating. This is a type of master recipe that you can use to customize with your favorite spices, fruits, herbs, and even veggies.

1. Preheat the oven to 350°F.

2. Line 12 cups of a standard muffin tin with paper liners.

3. In a large bowl, gently whisk together the almond flour, baking soda, and salt.

4. In a medium bowl, whisk together the eggs, applesauce, agave nectar, coconut oil, vinegar, and vanilla.

5. Add the egg mixture to the flour mixture and stir until blended. Fold in the fresh fruit (if using).

6. Divide the batter evenly among the 12 muffin cups in the prepared pan.

7. Bake for 15 to 20 minutes, until the muffins are set at the centers and golden brown on the edges. Transfer to a cooling rack and let cool completely.

8. Store the muffins in a covered container in the refrigerator for up to 1 week or in the freezer for up to 3 months.

INGREDIENT TIP: *Any type of berry would be a nutritious add-in, especially blueberries and cherries, both of which are high in beneficial antioxidants and phytochemicals. For a savory version, mix in ½ cup of nutritional yeast and herbs such as basil or dill.*

PER SERVING: CALORIES: 80; CARBS: 3G; GLYCEMIC LOAD: 2; FIBER: 0G; SODIUM: 217MG; PROTEIN: 3G; FAT: 6G; SATURATED FAT: 2G

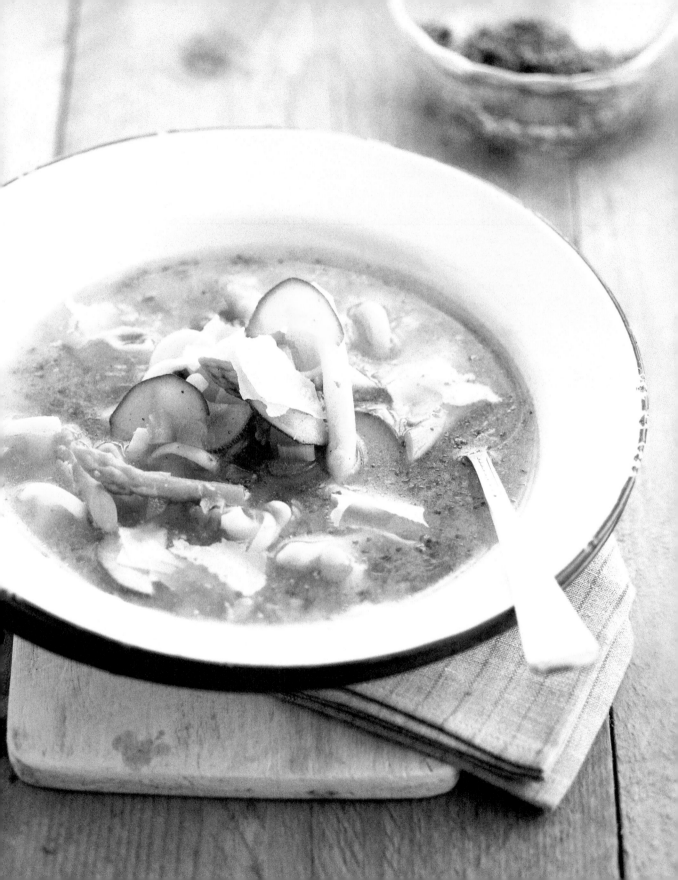

Soups and Salads

Spring Vegetable Soup

FERTILITY BOOST, LOWER CALORIE, GLUTEN FREE

2 tablespoons extra-virgin
  olive oil, divided
2 medium carrots, peeled
  and diced
1 large leek, trimmed,
  cleaned, and chopped
1 red bell pepper, diced
1 large celery stalk, diced
2 garlic cloves, minced
5 cups low-sodium
  vegetable broth
1 cup frozen peas
10 asparagus spears,
  cut into 1-inch pieces
1 medium zucchini,
  cut into ¼-inch slices
1 (15-ounce) can cannellini
  beans, drained and rinsed
1 teaspoon chopped fresh
  thyme, plus 1 tablespoon
  (optional)
¼ cup torn fresh basil
shaved Parmesan cheese
  (optional for garnish)
½ teaspoon salt
½ teaspoon freshly ground
  black pepper

SERVES 4 | PREP TIME: 15 MINUTES | COOK TIME: 30 MINUTES

This soup showcases a bounty of fresh veggies at the height of their season. Folate-rich asparagus and spinach team up with protein- and fiber-rich beans. Fresh herbs make this a perfect light and healthy meal option with a low glycemic index. This recipe is adaptable, so you can substitute your favorite vegetables. Serve this soup with sprouted whole grain bread for a nourishing and satisfying meal.

1. Heat a large soup pot or Dutch oven over medium heat. Add 1 tablespoon of the olive oil and swirl to coat. Add the carrots, leek, bell pepper, and celery, stir, and cook, stirring occasionally, for 5 minutes. Add the garlic and cook, stirring, for 1 minute. Increase the heat to high, add the broth, bring the liquid to a boil, then reduce the heat to low and simmer for 5 minutes.

2. Stir in the peas, asparagus, zucchini, and beans. Simmer until the asparagus is crisp tender, 3 to 4 minutes. Add the 1 teaspoon of thyme, and the basil, and stir, cooking for an additional minute.

3. Serve immediately, topped with the remaining tablespoon thyme and Parmesan cheese (if using). Season with the salt and pepper.

INGREDIENT TIP: *When choosing asparagus, look for stalks with tight tips and small leaves. The skin on the spears shouldn't be wrinkled, which is a sign they are dried out. Look for thinner spears, which are less fibrous, but remember they will cook faster.*

PER SERVING: CALORIES: 278; CARBS: 42G; GLYCEMIC LOAD: 14; FIBER: 11G; SODIUM: 765MG; PROTEIN: 12G; FAT: 8G; SATURATED FAT: 1G

Mushroom Barley Soup

FERTILITY BOOST, LOWER CALORIE, INFLAMMATION FIGHTER, DAIRY FREE, GLUTEN FREE

1 tablespoon olive oil

1 Vidalia onion, thinly sliced

Salt

8 ounces cremini mushrooms, sliced ¼ inch thick

2 large portobello mushrooms, cubed

1 large carrot, peeled and diced

1 medium zucchini, sliced into ¼-inch-thick half moons

1 garlic clove, minced

3 celery stalks, thinly sliced

1 large tomato, diced

¾ cups uncooked pearled barley

6 cups low-sodium vegetable broth

Freshly ground black pepper

3 tablespoons chopped fresh rosemary leaves, divided

3 tablespoons chopped fresh thyme, divided

INGREDIENT TIP: *You can vary the types of mushrooms used in this recipe or create a custom mix based on your preference. Shiitake, oyster, enoki, chanterelle, and button mushrooms are all rich in nutrients. You could also add a can of drained and rinsed beans to make the soup higher in protein.*

SERVES 4 | PREP TIME: 10 MINUTES | COOK TIME: 35 MINUTES

Many women with PCOS don't get enough vitamin D, which is essential for fertility and bone health. Up to 85 percent of women could have a vitamin D deficiency (Thomson, 2012). You can boost your intake by eating this rich and delicious soup. Mushrooms have many health benefits, including satiating and cholesterol-lowering fiber, vitamins, minerals, phytochemicals, and antioxidants. Eating mushrooms may also improve blood sugar and insulin levels.

1. Preheat a 4-quart pot over medium heat. Add the olive oil, onion, and a pinch of salt, and sauté until the onion is softened and translucent, about 5 minutes.

2. Add the mushrooms, carrot, and zucchini, and sauté until the vegetables are slightly softened and some of the moisture has been released, about 5 minutes. Mix in the garlic and sauté for 1 to 2 minutes.

3. Add the celery, tomato, barley, and broth, and season with salt and pepper. Cover and bring the liquid to a boil. Once it's boiling, reduce the heat to low. Stir in 2 tablespoons of the rosemary and 2 tablespoons of the thyme, and return the lid to the pot.

4. Simmer until the barley is tender, about 10 minutes. Taste the soup and season again with salt and pepper as desired. For best results, let the soup sit, covered, for at least 10 minutes so the flavors can blend.

5. Serve the soup garnished with the remaining tablespoons of rosemary and thyme.

PER SERVING: CALORIES: 213; CARBS: 38G; GLYCEMIC LOAD: 16; FIBER: 8G; SODIUM: 902MG; PROTEIN: 8G; FAT: 5G; SATURATED FAT: 1G

Creamy Vegan Kale Soup

INFLAMMATION FIGHTER, DAIRY FREE, GLUTEN FREE

2 tablespoons olive oil

1 medium leek, white and
light green parts only,
cleaned and sliced

4 garlic cloves, minced

8 cups low-sodium
vegetable broth

2 large bunches curly kale,
stemmed

1 cup raw cashews, soaked
in water for 4 to 8 hours,
drained and rinsed

4 sprigs fresh rosemary

4 sprigs fresh thyme

2 teaspoons ground nutmeg

2 tablespoons white
wine vinegar

¼ teaspoon salt

¼ teaspoon freshly ground
black pepper

¼ cup roasted pepitas
(shelled pumpkin seeds),
for garnish

FERTILITY BOOST TIP: *While this soup is already rich in vitamins C and E, folate, and antioxidants, you can increase the folate even further by adding another one or two vegetables. Some of the best vegetable choices are dark leafy greens (spinach, collard greens), asparagus, broccoli, and lentils.*

SERVES 4 | PREP TIME: 15 MINUTES, PLUS 4 TO 8 HOURS
SOAKING TIME | COOK TIME: 30 MINUTES

One of the most nutritious vegetables, kale provides antioxidants shown to reduce chronic inflammation and oxidative stress. Its good amounts of heart-healthy fiber omega-3 fatty acids can reduce inflammation. The creamy, buttery taste of this dish comes from vitamin E–rich cashews. For an extra dose of protein, enjoy it topped with crunchy pepitas.

1. Heat the oil in a large Dutch oven over medium heat. Add the leek and garlic and sauté until softened, about 5 minutes. Stir in the broth and remove the pot from the heat.

2. Working in batches, put the kale leaves into a food processor (or blender) and pulse until very finely chopped. Transfer to the pot with the broth.

3. Put the cashews in the food processor (or blender). Blend until smooth, stopping to scrape down the sides of the bowl with a spatula as needed.

4. Transfer the cashew mixture to the pot with the kale and broth, and stir in the rosemary, thyme, and nutmeg. Place the pot over high heat and bring the liquid to a low boil. Reduce the heat to medium low and simmer, uncovered, until the kale is tender, about 10 minutes.

5. Stir in the vinegar, salt, and pepper. Taste and adjust the seasonings as desired.

6. Ladle into bowls and garnish with the pepitas.

PER SERVING: CALORIES: 371; CARBS: 34G; GLYCEMIC LOAD: 11; FIBER: 4G; SODIUM: 829MG; PROTEIN: 12G; FAT: 24G; SATURATED FAT: 4G

Roasted Red Pepper and White Bean Soup

FERTILITY BOOST, INFLAMMATION FIGHTER, DAIRY FREE, GLUTEN FREE

1 tablespoon extra-virgin olive oil, plus more for garnish
1 large white onion, diced
3 garlic cloves, mined
4 medium carrots, peeled and chopped
4 cups low-sodium vegetable broth
1 (12-ounce) jar roasted red bell peppers, drained and sliced thin, reserving some for garnish
1 (15-ounce) can cannellini beans, drained and rinsed
1 teaspoon dried basil
½ teaspoon dried thyme
2 teaspoons paprika
½ teaspoon salt
¼ cup tahini (sesame paste)

LOWER CALORIE TIP: *The tahini adds extra touch of richness to the soup, but you could substitute unsweetened almond or coconut milk (not canned) if you prefer, or omit it entirely. The soup will taste just as delicious with a lower calorie count.*

SERVES 4 | PREP TIME: 10 MINUTES | COOK TIME: 30 MINUTES

The decadent, almost sweet flavor of this soup comes from the roasted red bell peppers. Peppers are packed with vitamins A and C, folate, vitamin K, antioxidants, minerals, and fiber. Rich in antioxidants, peppers can lower the likelihood of chronic oxidative stress and excessive inflammation.

1. Heat the olive oil in a large soup pot over medium heat. Add the onion and garlic and sauté for about 3 minutes, until the onion begins to soften.

2. Add the carrots and sauté for 3 minutes.

3. Add the broth, bell peppers, beans, basil, thyme, paprika, and salt. Increase the heat to high, bring the liquid to a boil, then reduce the heat to low and simmer for 10 to 15 minutes, until the carrots are fork tender.

4. Stir in the tahini, increase the heat to high, bring the soup to a boil, and then immediately remove the pot from the heat.

5. Carefully pour the soup into a blender and purée until smooth.

6. Return the soup to the pot over high heat, and reheat if needed.

7. Ladle the soup into 4 bowls and garnish with a few drizzles of olive oil and a few of the reserved slices of roasted red peppers.

PER SERVING: CALORIES: 312; CARBS: 42G; GLYCEMIC LOAD: 14; FIBER: 9G; SODIUM: 714MG; PROTEIN: 12G; FAT: 12G; SATURATED FAT: 2G

Tuscan Vegetable Soup

FERTILITY BOOST, LOWER CALORIE, DAIRY FREE, GLUTEN FREE

1½ cups peeled and
   cubed eggplant
1 cup water
1 (14.5-ounce) can
   no-salt-added diced
   tomatoes with their juice
½ cup sliced button
   mushrooms
1 portobello
   mushroom, cubed
1 garlic clove, minced
1 cup chopped zucchini
1 tablespoon chopped
   fresh thyme
   (or 1 teaspoon dried)
1 tablespoon chopped fresh
   sage (or ½ teaspoon dried)
Salt
Freshly ground black pepper
2 packed cups baby
   spinach leaves

SERVES 4 | PREP TIME: 15 MINUTES | COOK TIME: 25 MINUTES

Once thought to have no nutritional merit, the misunderstood eggplant is loaded with health benefits. Low in calories, this purple vegetable can aid in weight management and blood sugar control because of its high fiber content. It is also a great source of phytonutrients, folate, potassium, magnesium, and vitamins C and B_6, which benefit heart health, pregnancy, bone health, and digestion.

1. In a 3-quart saucepan over high heat, combine the eggplant, water, tomatoes with their juice, button mushrooms, portobello mushroom, garlic, zucchini, thyme, and sage, and season with salt and pepper. Bring to a boil. Cover the pot, reduce the heat to low, and simmer for 20 minutes.

2. Add the spinach and simmer, covered, for an additional 5 minutes or until the vegetables are tender.

3. Ladle into 4 bowls and serve hot.

INFLAMMATION FIGHTER TIP: *You can increase the inflammatory power of this soup by adding 1 cup of chopped celery, a veggie shown to help improve blood pressure and cholesterol and reduce inflammation in the body. For a truly anti-inflammatory meal, serve this soup as a starter preceding an entrée of grilled salmon.*

PER SERVING: CALORIES: 42; CARBS: 8G; GLYCEMIC LOAD: 3; FIBER: 3G; SODIUM: 51MG; PROTEIN: 3G; FAT: 1G; SATURATED FAT: 0G

Black Bean and Chickpea Veggie Chili

INFLAMMATION FIGHTER, DAIRY FREE, GLUTEN FREE

2 tablespoons olive oil

1 large white onion, chopped

Salt

Freshly ground black pepper

2 garlic cloves, minced

1 medium green
bell pepper, diced

2 celery stalks, chopped

1 (14.5-ounce) can diced
fire-roasted tomatoes and
their juice

1 (15-ounce) can black beans,
drained and rinsed

1 (15-ounce) can chickpeas
(garbanzo beans), drained
and rinsed

2 teaspoons ground cumin

1½ teaspoons
smoked paprika

1 teaspoon dried oregano

2 tablespoons chili powder

2 cups stemmed and
chopped kale

Juice of ½ lime

1 green onion (white and
light green parts only),
chopped, for garnish

½ lime, cut into 4 slices,
for garnish

1 avocado, sliced, for garnish

SERVES 4 | PREP TIME: 10 MINUTES | COOK TIME: 35 MINUTES

The smoky, complex flavors of this simple chili come from basic pantry ingredients, vegetables, and spices. Beans are an excellent food to include in an anti-inflammatory diet because of their low glycemic index and high fiber and anti-oxidant content. Include them in your diet as often as you can for long lasting, plant-powered energy.

1. Heat the olive oil in a large soup pot over medium heat. Add the onion, season with salt and pepper, and stir. Sauté until the onion is slightly translucent, about 3 minutes. Then add the garlic, green bell pepper, and celery. Sauté until soft, 5 to 8 minutes. (Turn the heat down to low if the garlic gets too brown.)

2. Add the canned tomatoes and their juice, then fill the can with water and add it to the pot. Stir to combine. Add the beans, chickpeas, cumin, paprika, oregano, chili powder, and kale, and season with salt and pepper. Cover, reduce the heat to low, and cook for 25 minutes, stirring occasionally.

3. Stir in the lime juice.

4. Ladle the chili into 4 bowls and garnish with the green onion, lime slices, and avocado slices.

FERTILITY BOOST TIP: *For additional fertility and pregnancy support, add 1 cup of choline-rich cauliflower florets, 1 cup of vitamin D–rich sliced button mushrooms, and top with a tablespoon of chopped walnuts, which contain high amounts of omega-3 fatty acids.*

PER SERVING: CALORIES: 491; CARBS: 71G; GLYCEMIC LOAD: 25; FIBER: 23G; SODIUM: 89MG; PROTEIN: 22G; FAT: 16G; SATURATED FAT: 2G

Miso Tofu Soup

FERTILITY BOOST, LOWER CALORIE, DAIRY FREE, GLUTEN FREE

5 cups water

1 sheet nori (dried seaweed), cut into large rectangles (optional)

½ cup chopped green onion (white and light green parts)

1 tablespoon peeled and grated fresh ginger

1 garlic clove, thinly sliced

4 tablespoons white miso paste

1 cup chopped green Swiss chard leaves

6 ounces firm tofu, drained and cut into ½-inch cubes

SERVES 4 | PREP TIME: 5 MINUTES | COOK TIME: 15 MINUTES

This comforting soup is brimming with soy, an excellent source of plant-based protein and antioxidants, and nori, a seaweed superfood high in essential minerals that can help maintain healthy blood sugar levels and support a healthy pregnancy. Chard adds a serving of green vegetables along with fertility-boosting nutrients, such as vitamins A and C, folic acid, calcium, and iron.

1. Bring the water to a boil in a 4-quart pot over medium-high heat. Add the nori (if using), green onion, ginger, and garlic. Reduce the heat to low, cover, and simmer for 10 minutes.

2. In a small bowl, put the miso paste, add a few drops hot water, and whisk until smooth. Stir into the soup.

3. Add the chard and tofu to the pot, return the soup to a gentle simmer, and simmer until the chard is tender, about 5 minutes.

4. Serve immediately.

INFLAMMATION FIGHTER TIP: *Dulse, kelp, wakame, agar agar, nori, and other sea vegetables are some of the most mineral-rich foods on the planet. Containing high amounts of magnesium, potassium, iodine, and vitamins A, C, and K, these vegetables provide excellent anti-inflammatory healing benefits. They make great additions to soups and salads and can replace the need for added salt.*

PER SERVING: CALORIES: 88; CARBS: 9G; GLYCEMIC LOAD: 4; FIBER: 2G; SODIUM: 751MG; PROTEIN: 9G; FAT: 3G; SATURATED FAT: 1G

Almond Chicken and Greens Soup

INFLAMMATION FIGHTER, DAIRY FREE, GLUTEN FREE

4 cups low-sodium
   chicken broth
½ small yellow onion, diced
2 garlic cloves, minced
1 red bell pepper, diced
1 large sweet potato, peeled
   and diced
8 ounces boneless, skinless
   chicken breast, cut into
   bite-size pieces
½ cup natural creamy
   almond butter
2 cups stemmed and thinly
   sliced kale
2 tablespoons peeled and
   minced fresh ginger
Salt
Freshly ground black pepper
1 lime, cut into 4 wedges

SERVES 4 | PREP TIME: 10 MINUTES | COOK TIME: 30 MINUTES

Almond butter creates a slightly creamy texture and rich flavor in this high-protein chicken soup, without the use of butter or cream. Almonds contain impressive amounts of magnesium, which can reduce blood sugar and maintain healthy cholesterol levels. They are also a good source of vitamin E and provide plant-powered protein. Enjoy this with a side salad of mixed baby greens.

1. In a 4-quart pot over medium-high heat, combine the broth, onion, garlic, bell pepper, and sweet potato and bring to a boil. Reduce the heat to low. Add the chicken, cover, and simmer for 20 minutes or until the chicken is cooked through.

2. In a small bowl, whisk together the almond butter and ½ cup of the soup mixture into a thick paste. Set aside.

3. Add the kale and ginger to the soup, and stir to combine. Increase the heat to high and bring the liquid to a boil; then reduce the heat to low and simmer, covered, for 5 minutes. Stir in the almond butter paste and season with salt and pepper.

4. Ladle the soup into 4 soup bowls and squeeze each with a lime wedge.

INGREDIENT TIP: *You can substitute cubed butternut squash for the sweet potato or replace it entirely with a type of cooked bean for added protein. Lentils would make a good choice: they cook in 20 minutes or less, so they could be added to the pot with the chicken.*

PER SERVING: CALORIES: 421; CARBS: 32G; GLYCEMIC LOAD: 9; FIBER: 4G; SODIUM: 841MG; PROTEIN: 15G; FAT: 28G; SATURATED FAT: 4G

Vegetable Quinoa Mega Bowl

INFLAMMATION FIGHTER, DAIRY FREE, GLUTEN FREE

FOR THE DRESSING

⅓ cup natural almond butter

⅓ cup extra-virgin olive oil

3 garlic cloves, minced
  (approximately
  1 tablespoon)

3-inch piece fresh ginger,
  peeled and minced
  (1 to 2 tablespoons)

Juice of 3 limes
  (approximately ⅓ cup)

Water, to thin

**FOR THE VEGETABLE
QUINOA**

1 cup uncooked quinoa
  (see Ingredient Tip,
  page 56)

2 cups water

½ head red cabbage,
  shredded (approximately
  3 cups)

½ cup diced green onions

½ cup fresh cilantro, chopped

1 (15-ounce) can navy beans,
  drained and rinsed

1 cup diced zucchini

¾ cup chopped almonds

FERTILITY BOOST TIP: *For
added vitamin D, omega-3 fatty
acids, and high-quality protein,
add a chopped hard-boiled
egg. Women with PCOS who
eat foods containing omega-3
fatty acids on a weekly basis
have been found to experience
improved fertility.*

SERVES 6 | PREP TIME: 25 MINUTES | COOK TIME: 20 MINUTES

*If you need a dish that will fill you up without weighing you
down, look no further than this colorful mega bowl, with
protein-packed, low-GI quinoa, crunchy red cabbage and
veggies, heart-healthy, high-fiber navy beans, and a dressing
made with vitamin E–rich almond butter.*

TO MAKE THE DRESSING

Put all of the ingredients in a food processor (or blender)
and blend until smooth. Add water, a few drops at a
time, as needed to thin until desired consistency.

TO MAKE THE VEGETABLE QUINOA

1. In a medium saucepan over medium-high heat,
combine the quinoa and the water. Bring to a rolling boil
and let it cook for 1 minute; then reduce the heat to low,
cover the pan, and cook for 15 minutes, until the quinoa
absorbs the water.

2. Remove the pan from the heat and let it stand
for 5 minutes, covered. Remove the lid and fluff gently
with a fork. Transfer to a large mixing bowl.

3. Add the cabbage, green onions, cilantro, beans,
zucchini, and almonds, and stir to combine. Pour the
dressing over the quinoa-veggie mixture and toss until
the ingredients are all well coated.

4. Distribute into 6 bowls and serve immediately.
Or place in an airtight container and refrigerate for
up to 3 days.

PER SERVING: CALORIES: 533; CARBS: 50G; GLYCEMIC LOAD: 18;
FIBER: 15G; SODIUM: 21MG; PROTEIN: 19G; FAT: 31G; SATURATED FAT: 3G

Broccoli Sprouts Salad with Walnuts and Blueberries

LOWER CALORIE, INFLAMMATION FIGHTER, DAIRY FREE, GLUTEN FREE

2 cups loosely packed fresh
    broccoli sprouts
1 cup chopped kale leaves
1 cup chopped collard
    green leaves
½ cup chopped walnuts
½ cup fresh blueberries
Handful fresh cilantro,
    chopped
1 tablespoon extra-virgin
    olive oil
Salt
Freshly ground black pepper

SERVES 4 | PREP TIME: 5 MINUTES

Broccoli sprouts are the immature versions of the broccoli plant with a bonus: these young sprouts contain up to 50 times more of the antioxidant sulforaphane than mature broccoli contains, boosting their health benefits and free radical–fighting potential. Sprouts are featured in this recipe with other nutritional powerhouses, including omega-3–rich walnuts, anthocyanidin-rich blueberries, and kale and collards, which contain impressive amounts of vitamin C and K, folate, and fiber. Prepared in minutes, this light and tasty salad makes a great starter dish.

1. In a large bowl, combine the sprouts, kale, and collard greens.

2. Add the walnuts, blueberries, cilantro, and olive oil and toss to combine.

3. Season with salt and pepper. Serve immediately.

INGREDIENT TIP: *It is super easy to grow your own sprouts at home by using a mason jar and sprouting lid. You simply choose the seeds you want to sprout, place them in the jar with some water, and soak them overnight. Drain the water the next morning and rinse them well. Lay the jar on its side in indirect sunlight. Continue rinsing and draining once a day until your sprouts are ready.*

PER SERVING: CALORIES: 222; CARBS: 23G; GLYCEMIC LOAD: 9; FIBER: 2G; SODIUM: 46MG; PROTEIN: 8G; FAT: 14G; SATURATED FAT: 1G

Mason Jar Taco Salad

FERTILITY BOOST, DAIRY FREE, GLUTEN FREE

1 tablespoon extra-virgin
   olive oil, divided
6 ounces boneless skinless
   chicken breast, cut into
   bite-size pieces
1 large red bell pepper,
   seeded and sliced
½ large white onion,
   roughly chopped
2 teaspoons minced garlic
2 teaspoons cumin seeds
½ cup canned black beans,
   drained and rinsed
Pinch salt
1 medium avocado, pitted
   and cubed
Juice of 1 large lime
4 Roma tomatoes, chopped
½ cucumber, peeled
   and chopped
½ cup chopped fresh cilantro
2 cups baby spinach leaves

SERVES 2 | PREP TIME: 10 MINUTES | COOK TIME: 20 MINUTES

You can feel good knowing you are packing both a nutritious and earth-friendly lunch when you prepare this mason jar taco salad. Chicken breast adds lean protein to keep you feeling full, and the mix of vegetables provides an array of nutrients, including vitamins A, C, K, and E and the minerals calcium and iron. Avocado and olive oil add healthy fats, and the beans add plant protein, fiber, and folate. Because the salad is strategically layered to prevent the ingredients from getting soggy, you can make it ahead, bring it to work, and then empty the contents into a bowl at lunchtime. You will need two wide-mouth quart-size mason jars for this salad.

1. In a large skillet, heat ½ tablespoon of the olive oil over medium-high heat. Add the chicken breast and sauté until golden brown, about 8 minutes. Transfer to a small bowl.

2. Add the remaining ½ tablespoon olive oil to the skillet and reduce the heat to medium. Add the bell pepper, onion, and garlic, and sauté until softened and browned, about 5 minutes.

3. In a small, dry pan over medium-high heat, add the cumin seeds, and toast, stirring frequently, until golden brown and fragrant, about 2 minutes. Transfer to a cutting board and crush with the bottom of a sturdy glass.

4. Add the crushed cumin seeds and black beans to the skillet with the veggies, and stir in the salt. Remove the skillet from the heat.

5. Put the avocado and lime juice into a small bowl. Using a fork, mash them together until smooth.

6. To assemble the salads in the mason jars, spread one-fourth of the chopped tomatoes evenly in the bottom of each jar. Put one-fourth of the avocado-lime mixture on top of each, and gently spread out. In each jar, spread a layer of the cumin and roasted veggies, followed by a layer of chicken. Add one-fourth of the remaining tomatoes to each jar, and then add a layer of cucumbers. Finish by adding ¼ cup of the cilantro to each, topped by as much of the spinach as possible.

7. Seal and refrigerate. To eat, turn the jar over and shake to distribute the ingredients. Eat out of the jar, or pour onto a plate.

COOKING TIP: *Set aside time on a Sunday to prepare enough mason jar salads for your week of lunches. Use leftover grains, beans, roasted veggies, nuts, and seeds and simply follow this layering formula so that the ingredients stay separated just enough to avoid getting soggy: first pour in the dressing, then add vegetables and/or fruits, grains and/or beans, crunchy nuts and seeds, and finish it off with the leafy greens.*

PER SERVING: CALORIES: 524; CARBS: 44G; GLYCEMIC LOAD: 16; FIBER: 14G; SODIUM: 469MG; PROTEIN: 21G; FAT: 31G; SATURATED FAT: 5G

Chickpea, Tomato, and Basil Salad

LOWER CALORIE, INFLAMMATION FIGHTER, DAIRY FREE, GLUTEN FREE

1 (15-ounce) can chickpeas (garbanzo beans), drained and rinsed

1 pint cherry tomatoes, halved

1 cup chopped fresh basil leaves

4 garlic cloves, minced

1 tablespoon red wine vinegar

1 tablespoon apple cider vinegar

2 teaspoons extra-virgin olive oil

½ tablespoon honey

Pinch salt

Freshly ground black pepper

SERVES 2 TO 4 | PREP TIME: 10 MINUTES, PLUS 20 MINUTES TO CHILL

This flavorful salad is quick to prepare and loaded with nutrients from the tomatoes, chickpeas, and fresh basil. Tomatoes contain all four major carotenoids—alpha- and beta-carotene, lutein, and lycopene—which individually have benefits but together act synergistically, boosting their antioxidant activity even further. The volatile oils in basil can reduce inflammation in the body, making this herb an excellent choice for managing PCOS. With added staying power from the high-fiber, high-protein chickpeas, this salad makes a satisfying side dish or light lunch.

In a medium bowl, mix together all the ingredients. Chill for about 20 minutes before serving.

INFLAMMATION FIGHTER TIP: *Tomatoes and olive oil are two of the most anti-inflammatory foods available, but you can also add several other ingredients that work well in this dish. For example, to add kale, remove the stems from 1 bunch of green kale, rub the leaves with some olive oil or avocado to soften, then chop them and add to the salad. Kale's combination of 45 flavonoids gives it a leading dietary role in avoiding chronic inflammation and oxidative stress.*

PER SERVING: CALORIES: 676; CARBS:134G; GLYCEMIC LOAD: 67; FIBER: 18G; SODIUM: 75MG; PROTEIN: 21G; FAT: 10G; SATURATED FAT: 1G

Asian Peanut Slaw

INFLAMMATION FIGHTER, DAIRY FREE, GLUTEN FREE

1 (12-ounce) bag non-GMO
   frozen shelled edamame
3 cups shredded
   green cabbage
2 cups shredded carrots
1 cup shredded
   purple cabbage
1 cup chopped fresh cilantro
1 cup green onions,
   chopped (white and light
   green parts)
1 cup roasted
   unsalted peanuts
⅓ cup extra-virgin olive oil
3 tablespoons rice vinegar
1 tablespoon sesame oil
1 teaspoon Bragg's
   liquid aminos
1 teaspoon ground ginger
1 teaspoon honey

SERVES 6 | PREP TIME: 10 MINUTES | COOK TIME: 10 MINUTES

This Asian-inspired, nutrient-rich salad makes a super quick lunch, easy side dish, or tasty light dinner. Edamame, or green soybeans, is one of the only plant foods that is a complete protein, meaning that it has all of the required amino acids. It is also low in fat and contains essential fatty acids, numerous vitamins, minerals, and fiber. Research on the use of soy in women with PCOS is overwhelmingly favorable for its use in improving metabolic aspects, reducing insulin, bad cholesterol, inflammatory markers, oxidative stress, and testosterone (Grassi, 2016).

1. Place the edamame in a medium saucepan over medium-high heat, cover with water, and cook until tender, about 8 minutes. Drain in a colander.

2. Meanwhile, in a large bowl, combine the green cabbage, carrots, purple cabbage, cilantro, green onions, and peanuts.

3. In a small bowl, whisk together the olive oil, rice vinegar, sesame oil, aminos, ginger, and honey until the mixture is emulsified.

4. Add the dressing and cooked edamame to the cabbage mixture and toss until thoroughly combined.

5. Serve immediately.

COOKING TIP: *This salad can be prepared in minutes by using prechopped cabbage and carrots. Keep a bag or two of frozen edamame on hand for use as a quick snack, a smoothie ingredient, to make hummus, or as a wrap filling.*

PER SERVING: CALORIES: 378; CARBS: 21G; GLYCEMIC LOAD: 5; FIBER: 8G; SODIUM: 103MG; PROTEIN: 11G; FAT: 30G; SATURATED FAT: 4G

Moroccan Spiced Buckwheat Salad

INFLAMMATION FIGHTER, DAIRY TREE, GLUTEN FREE

2 cups cooked buckwheat

1 (15-ounce) can chickpeas (garbanzo beans), drained and rinsed

1 small red onion, chopped

2 cups stemmed, thinly sliced kale

1 cup chopped carrots

4 dried apricots, finely chopped

2 green onions, sliced (white and light green parts)

¼ cup chopped fresh cilantro

2 tablespoons extra-virgin olive oil

⅓ cup rice wine vinegar

3 teaspoons ground cumin

½ teaspoon salt

¼ cup sunflower seeds (optional)

SERVES 4 | PREP TIME: 10 MINUTES

Despite its name, buckwheat is a gluten-free grain alternative loaded with health benefits, especially for women with PCOS. Similar to a whole grain, it is a great source of heart-healthy fiber and protein, which keep you feeling full longer. Buckwheat has a low glycemic load and is a good source of fatigue-fighting iron, bone-healthy calcium, and phytochemicals. It also contains both omega-3 and omega-6 fatty acids. Low-GI apricots and antioxidant-rich cumin add Moroccan flair to this nutritious dish.

1. In a large bowl, stir together the buckwheat, chickpeas, red onion, kale, carrots, apricots, green onions, and cilantro.

2. In a small bowl, whisk the olive oil, vinegar, cumin, and salt until combined.

3. Add the dressing to the buckwheat and vegetable mixture, and toss until coated.

4. Serve topped with the sunflower seeds (if using).

FERTILITY BOOST TIP: *For added choline, a nutrient with the potential to reduce a harmful gene that may result in birth defects, add 2 cups cauliflower florets. The cauliflower will also add another vegetable serving to each portion, along with additional phytochemicals and antioxidants.*

PER SERVING: CALORIES: 359; CARBS: 56G; GLYCEMIC LOAD: 22; FIBER: 13G; SODIUM: 342MG; PROTEIN: 14G; FAT: 10G; SATURATED FAT: 1G

Persian Cucumber Salad

LOWER CALORIE, INFLAMMATION FIGHTER, DAIRY FREE, GLUTEN FREE

5 small Persian cucumbers, unpeeled, or 1 large English cucumber, peeled

1½ cups cherry tomatoes

½ small red onion

3 tablespoons coarsely chopped fresh flat-leaf parsley

2 tablespoons coarsely chopped fresh mint

1 tablespoon extra-virgin olive oil

3 tablespoons freshly squeezed lime juice

1 teaspoon freshly grated lime zest

⅓ teaspoon coarse sea salt

¼ teaspoon freshly ground black pepper

SERVES 4 | PREP TIME: 10 MINUTES, PLUS 10 MINUTES TO SIT (OR 2 HOURS TO CHILL)

This colorful, refreshing salad is a traditional side dish in Iran. It is made with Persian cucumbers tossed with a mild citrusy dressing. Very low in calories, this vegetable is a valuable source of antioxidants, including vitamin C, beta-carotene, and manganese. Persian cucumbers also contain numerous flavonoid antioxidants that act to reduce inflammation in the body by scavenging free radicals. Serve this light salad or side dish on a bed of julienned kale.

1. Dice the cucumbers, tomatoes, and red onion into small cubes and transfer them to a medium bowl.

2. Add the chopped parsley and mint.

3. In a small bowl, whisk together the olive oil, lime juice, lime zest, salt, pepper, and olive oil.

4. Add the dressing to the salad ingredients and toss gently to coat. Let the salad sit at room temperature for 10 minutes so the flavors can mingle, or cover the bowl and refrigerate for up to 2 hours.

5. Serve chilled.

INGREDIENT TIP: *Persian cucumbers are nearly seedless and are thin-skinned enough to be eaten unpeeled. They are usually 5 to 6 inches long and can be used interchangeably with the similar but larger English cucumber.*

PER SERVING: CALORIES: 26; CARBS: 6G; GLYCEMIC LOAD: 2; FIBER: 1G; SODIUM: 297MG; PROTEIN: 1G; FAT: 0G; SATURATED FAT: 0G

Artichoke Millet Power Salad

INFLAMMATION FIGHTER, DAIRY FREE, GLUTEN FREE

2 tablespoons extra-virgin
olive oil, divided
2 medium shallots
1 garlic clove, minced
¼ teaspoon salt
½ teaspoon freshly ground
black pepper
⅓ cup uncooked millet
⅔ cup water
1 cup finely chopped fresh
flat-leaf parsley
¼ cup freshly squeezed
lemon juice
2 tablespoons
balsamic vinegar
1 pint cherry
tomatoes, halved
2 small zucchini, trimmed
and chopped
1 (15-ounce) can cannellini
beans, drained and rinsed
1 (15-ounce) can artichoke
hearts in water, drained
and quartered
½ cup roasted pepitas
(shelled pumpkin seeds),
for garnish

SERVES 4 | PREP TIME: 10 MINUTES | COOK TIME: 20 MINUTES, PLUS 10 MINUTES (OR UP TO 2 HOURS) TO CHILL

Millet is an ancient seed, originally hailing from Africa and northern China, with a creamy consistency similar to mashed potatoes or fluffy rice. A gluten-free grain alternative, millet is a good source of magnesium, which is essential for keeping a healthy heartbeat, sustaining immune function, and managing inflammation. In this salad, it is combined with artichokes, zucchini, tomatoes, and pepitas (shelled pumpkin seeds) to create a nutritious masterpiece that will provide you with hours of steady energy.

1. Heat 1 tablespoon of the olive oil in a small saucepan over medium heat. Add the shallots, garlic, salt, and pepper, and sauté until soft and translucent, about 5 minutes.

2. Increase the heat to high and add the millet. While stirring constantly, allow the millet to brown slightly, about 3 minutes.

3. Add the water and bring to a boil. Then reduce the heat to low, cover, and simmer for 10 minutes. Remove the pan from the heat and let the millet steam, covered, for 5 minutes. Transfer to a large bowl and fluff with a fork. Allow to cool slightly.

4. In a medium bowl, combine the chopped parsley, lemon juice, balsamic vinegar, and remaining 1 tablespoon of oil. Massage the mixture together to soften the parsley.

5. To the bowl with the millet mixture, add the tomatoes, zucchini, beans, and artichoke hearts. Add the parsley mixture, and toss until combined.

6. Cover and chill for 10 minutes or up to 2 hours before serving.

7. Serve garnished with the pepitas.

INGREDIENT TIP: *Millet makes a great breakfast porridge because of its creamy consistency. Just add fruit and nuts and serve it with a hard-boiled egg. Ground millet can also be added to muffin recipes for an extra boost of minerals and fiber.*

PER SERVING: CALORIES: 433; CARBS: 58G; GLYCEMIC LOAD: 22; FIBER: 19G; SODIUM: 226MG; PROTEIN: 19G; FAT: 16G; SATURATED FAT: 3G

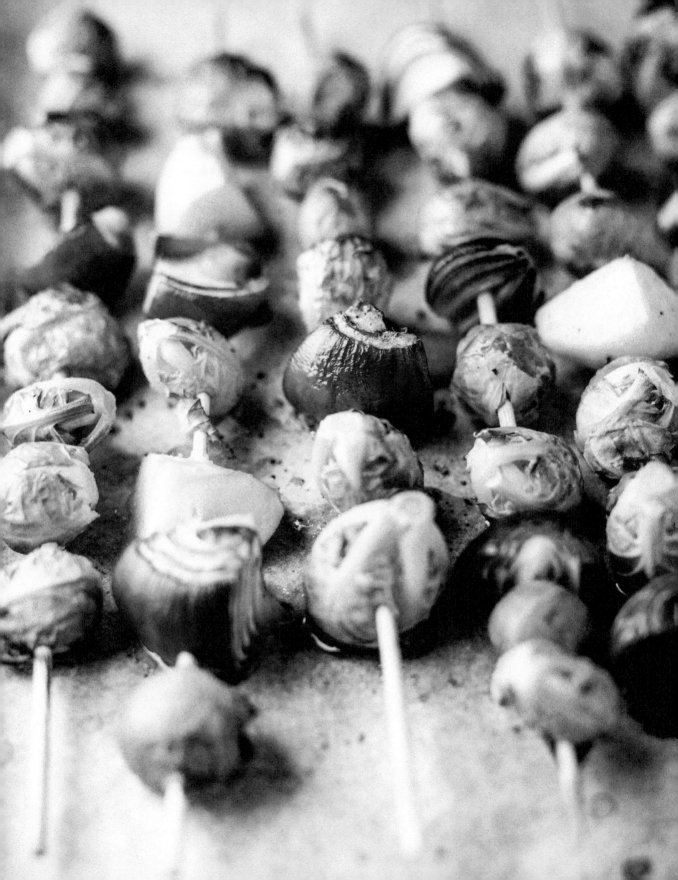

5

Snacks and Sides

Portable Paella Cups

INFLAMMATION FIGHTER, DAIRY FREE, GLUTEN FREE

1 cup water

¼ cup chickpea flour
(you can substitute
almond flour)

1 tablespoon olive oil

1 tablespoon flaxseed meal

2 garlic cloves, minced

¾ teaspoon ground turmeric

¾ teaspoon salt

2 cups cooked and cooled
brown rice

⅔ cup canned chickpeas
(garbanzo beans), drained
and rinsed

½ cup frozen
green peas, thawed

½ cup roasted red
peppers, chopped

⅓ cup artichoke hearts,
drained and chopped

SERVES 8 | PREP TIME: 20 MINUTES | COOK TIME: 30 MINUTES

Paella is a rice dish from eastern Spain traditionally prepared with whatever the cook has on hand. In this dish, readily available ingredients are used and antioxidant-rich turmeric takes the place of the more expensive saffron. Cooked in a muffin tin, these rice and bean cups are high in blood sugar–stabilizing protein and fiber, and best of all they are portable, making them a great on-the-go snack.

1. Preheat the oven to 350°F.

2. Line 8 cups of a standard muffin tin with paper liners.

3. In a large bowl, whisk together the water, chickpea flour, olive oil, flaxseed meal, garlic, turmeric, salt, and pepper until blended. Stir in the rice, chickpeas, peas, red peppers, and artichoke hearts. Mix thoroughly to combine.

4. Divide the mixture evenly among the prepared muffin cups.

5. Bake for 25 to 30 minutes until the centers feel set and tops appear golden and crispy.

6. Cool completely in the tin. Remove the paella cups.

7. Serve at room temperature, cold, or rewarmed in the microwave for 15 to 30 seconds.

INGREDIENT TIP: *Chickpea flour can be found in most grocery stores or ordered online, and is high in fiber and protein, lending a rich flavor to dishes. You can make your own hummus or falafel using the flour and it is a wonderful ingredient in gluten-free cooking. Look for Bob's Red Mill brand.*

PER SERVING: CALORIES: 128; CARBS: 21G; GLYCEMIC LOAD: 9; FIBER: 4G; SODIUM: 241MG; PROTEIN: 4G; FAT: 3G; SATURATED FAT: 0G

"Cheesy" Baked Spinach Chips

LOWER CALORIE, INFLAMMATION FIGHTER, DAIRY FREE

2 cups baby spinach

1 tablespoon olive oil

3 tablespoons nutritional yeast, divided

¼ teaspoon garlic powder

Salt

Freshly ground black pepper

INGREDIENT TIP: *For more of a cheesy flavor and additional healthy fats, put 2 tablespoons of cashews, 2 tablespoons of shelled sunflower seeds, and 2 tablespoons of nutritional yeast in a food processor (or blender) and blend until smooth. Combine the spinach with the olive oil and nut mixture and toss until the leaves are coated. Then follow the rest of the recipe.*

SERVES 4 | PREP TIME: 5 MINUTES | COOK TIME: 25 MINUTES

Veggie chips make a nutritious alternative to high-fat processed snacks, and can fit the bill when you are looking to satisfy that urge for crunch. While kale chips can be found in most supermarkets, not everyone likes the somewhat bitter taste. This recipe uses the milder and equally delicious spinach and tops them with dairy-free nutritional yeast for a snack high in vitamins, minerals, and phytochemicals with a dash of protein.

1. Preheat the oven to 325°F.

2. Line 2 baking sheets with parchment paper.

3. In a medium bowl, combine the spinach, olive oil, and 2 tablespoons of the nutritional yeast, and gently toss until all of the spinach leaves are coated.

4. Lay the spinach leaves in a single layer on the prepared baking sheets. Sprinkle with the garlic powder, salt, pepper, and the remaining 1 tablespoon nutritional yeast.

5. Bake for 12 minutes; then turn the oven off and leave the pans in the oven for an additional 5 minutes.

6. Remove the pans from the oven and let the spinach sit for 5 minutes more to crisp up.

7. Once completely cooled, store in an airtight bag for 2 to 3 days. The crispy texture will begin to fade after 24 hours, so enjoy these right after baking as possible.

PER SERVING: CALORIES: 51; CARBS: 3G; GLYCEMIC LOAD: 1; FIBER: 2G; SODIUM: 38MG; PROTEIN: 3G; FAT: 4G; SATURATED FAT: 0G

Lentil-Stuffed Avocado

INFLAMMATION FIGHTER, DAIRY FREE, GLUTEN FREE

½ cup dry lentils

1 tablespoon extra-virgin olive oil

1 small white onion, halved and sliced

2 garlic cloves, chopped

10 cherry tomatoes, halved

⅛ teaspoon smoked paprika

Salt

Freshly ground black pepper

2 large avocados

2 tablespoons chopped fresh cilantro (optional)

SERVES 4 | PREP TIME: 5 MINUTES | COOK TIME: 35 MINUTES

Avocados are one of those fruits to keep on hand at all times, not only because they are delicious and nutritious, but because they can be used in so many creative ways in cooking. Filled with satiating fiber and healthy fats, in this recipe, creamy avocados are stuffed with inflammation-fighting lentils to create a delicious, portable, protein-rich snack, side dish, or light entrée.

1. Bring 2 cups of water to a boil in a medium saucepan over high heat. Stir in the lentils, and cook for 15 minutes. Drain.

2. Meanwhile, in a medium saucepan over medium heat, add the onion and sauté until translucent, about 3 minutes. Add the garlic and sauté for 1 minute.

3. Add the tomatoes and smoked paprika, season with salt and pepper, and stir to combine. Simmer for 10 minutes, stirring frequently. Taste and adjust the seasoning for salt and pepper.

4. Add the lentils to the vegetable mixture, stir, and cook for 2 to 3 minutes.

5. Cut the avocados in half, and core. Put the halves on 4 plates. Top with the lentil mixture and top with the chopped cilantro (if using).

INGREDIENT TIP: *A great trick for choosing a good avocado is to pop the little button stem off of the top end of the avocado. If the skin under it is green, it's a good choice. If the skin under it is brown, it's past its prime.*

PER SERVING: CALORIES: 312; CARBS: 30G; GLYCEMIC LOAD: 12; FIBER: 12G; SODIUM: 33MG; PROTEIN: 10G; FAT: 19G; SATURATED FAT: 4G

Mushroom Hummus Dippers

FERTILITY BOOST, DAIRY FREE, GLUTEN FREE

3 cups baby bello or
  portobello mushrooms,
  sliced
⅓ cup olive oil,
  plus 2 tablespoons
Salt
Freshly ground black pepper
1 (15-ounce) can chickpeas
  (garbanzo beans), drained
  and rinsed
⅓ cup tahini (sesame paste)
2 garlic cloves, minced
Juice of 1 lemon
Water
1 tablespoon chopped fresh
  flat-leaf parsley

LOWER CALORIE TIP: *You
can make this lower in calories
by decreasing the tahini to
2 tablespoons, adding 2 tablespoons of almond milk, and
lightly spraying the mushrooms
with olive oil cooking spray
instead of drizzling with the
⅓ cup oil.*

SERVES 6 | PREP TIME: 10 MINUTES | COOK TIME: 15 MINUTES

*This spin on a traditional hummus recipe uses vitamin D–rich
portobello mushrooms. Mushrooms are a very low-calorie
food, yet they contain a small amount of protein and are a
good source of fiber, blood pressure–regulating potassium,
and B vitamins. Portion the hummus into 8-ounce mason
jars, put a handful of short vegetable sticks vertically in the
hummus, screw on the top, and put it in your gym bag or
purse for a healthy, easy, on-the-go snack. You will need
6 (1-cup) mason jars for this recipe.*

1. Preheat the oven to 425°F.

2. Line a baking sheet with aluminum foil.

3. Layer the sliced mushrooms on the prepared pan,
drizzle with ⅓ cup of the olive oil, and season with salt
and pepper. Roast for 15 minutes until browned, stirring
them halfway through. Set aside on a cooling rack.

4. In a food processor (or blender), add the remaining
2 tablespoons olive oil, chickpeas, tahini, garlic, and
lemon juice. Pulse for a few seconds, adding a few drops
of water as needed to thin the mixture. Add the mushrooms and pulse again, adding a few drops of water
until the desired consistency is reached. Season with
salt and pepper.

5. Portion into 6 mason jars or another airtight
container. Refrigerate for up to 4 days.

PER SERVING: CALORIES: 332; CARBS: 26G; GLYCEMIC LOAD: 9; FIBER: 8G;
SODIUM: 45MG; PROTEIN: 11G; FAT: 23G; SATURATED FAT: 2G

Real Food Vegan Protein Bars

GLUTEN FREE, DAIRY FREE

Olive oil cooking spray
½ cup old-fashioned
   rolled oats
2 tablespoons chia seeds
⅓ cup (about 8) dried
   apricots, roughly chopped
1¾ cups canned chickpeas
   (garbanzo beans), drained
   and rinsed
3 tablespoons honey
2 tablespoons hemp seeds
⅔ cup unsweetened almond
   or coconut milk
1 teaspoon vanilla extract
1 teaspoon ground cinnamon

SERVES 10 | PREP TIME: 10 MINUTES | COOK TIME: 30 MINUTES

Reaching for a packaged protein bar labeled "healthy" or "natural" may sound like a good idea, but the FDA doesn't regulate those words and there are no legal definitions. This means your natural-sounding bar may be highly processed. This recipe for homemade snack bars uses chickpeas, which help stabilize blood sugar, and healthy fats from chia and hemp seeds. Sweetness is provided by low glycemic index apricots.

1. Preheat the oven to 350°F.

2. Coat a 9-by-9-inch baking pan with olive oil cooking spray.

3. In a blender, combine the oats, chia seeds, and apricots, and blend until chopped. Pour into a large mixing bowl.

4. In the blender, add the chickpeas and blend until chopped but not puréed, with a texture similar to oatmeal. Add to the oats mixture.

5. To the oats mixture, add the honey, hemp seeds, almond milk, vanilla, and cinnamon and mix well.

6. Add the batter to the prepared pan and press down so it is even on top.

7. Bake for about 30 minutes, or until the edges are golden brown and the center is no longer soft.

8. Cool in the pan on a cooling rack. Cut into squares. Store in an airtight container in the refrigerator for up to 4 days, or in a resealable plastic bag in the freezer for up to 3 months.

INFLAMMATION FIGHTER TIP: *While the beans, seeds, and fruit used in this recipe all contain high levels of inflammation-fighting antioxidants, you can vary the recipe and substitute others that are just as nutritious depending on your preferences. Some good choices include dried blueberries or cherries, flaxseed meal, and pepitas (shelled pumpkin seeds), and you could use quinoa flakes in place of the oats.*

PER SERVING: CALORIES: 164; CARBS: 22G; GLYCEMIC LOAD: 10; FIBER: 4G; SODIUM: 5MG; PROTEIN: 6G; FAT: 7G; SATURATED FAT: 3G

Garlicky Roasted Edamame

LOWER CALORIE, INFLAMMATION FIGHTER, DAIRY FREE, GLUTEN FREE

Olive oil cooking spray
1 pound non-GMO frozen, shelled edamame, thawed
½ teaspoon salt
½ teaspoon freshly ground black pepper
½ teaspoon garlic powder
1½ teaspoons olive oil

MAKES ABOUT 22 (¼ CUP) SERVINGS | PREP TIME: 5 MINUTES
COOK TIME: 50 MINUTES

Green soybeans, otherwise known as edamame, are low in fat, rich in natural phytochemicals, vitamins, and minerals. Some of their health benefits include a stronger immune system, improved bone health, weight management, and improved cardiovascular health. Plus they are loaded with the perfect energy-boosting mix of slow digesting carbs, protein, and fiber. Prepare a batch of these and portion them into ¼-cup servings in small resealable plastic bags for a satiating portable snack.

1. Preheat the oven to 400°F.

2. Lightly coat a baking sheet with olive oil cooking spray.

3. In a medium bowl, toss the edamame with the salt, pepper, garlic, and olive oil.

4. Spread out on the prepared pan, and roast for 50 to 60 minutes or until golden brown.

5. Cool completely. Store in an airtight container at room temperature for up to 4 days.

INGREDIENT TIP: *You can vary the seasonings depending on your preferences. For a spicy twist, add a dash of cayenne pepper. For a sweet and salty mix, replace the garlic powder with stevia powder and add a dash of ground cinnamon.*

PER SERVING: CALORIES: 25; CARBS: 2G; GLYCEMIC LOAD: 1; FIBER: 1G; SODIUM: 54MG; PROTEIN: 2G; FAT: 1G; SATURATED FAT: 0G

No-Bake Mini Stuffed Peppers

LOWER CALORIE, INFLAMMATION FIGHTER, GLUTEN FREE

1 (24 to 32-ounce) bag mini bell peppers

1 (15-ounce) can chickpeas (garbanzo beans), drained and rinsed

¼ cup plain, unsweetened Greek yogurt

1 tablespoon apple cider vinegar

½ teaspoon mustard powder

½ teaspoon dried thyme

2 green onions, sliced thinly

½ teaspoon salt

Pinch cayenne pepper

MAKES 30 | PREP TIME: 20 MINUTES

Colorful, antioxidant-rich mini sweet peppers are filled with a high protein, blood sugar–stabilizing bean mixture to create a perfectly, portable snack. Peppers are very low in calories and high in vitamin C, phytochemicals, and carotenoids, which provide your body with antioxidant and anti-inflammatory benefits. This high-powered snack doesn't require baking, has minimal ingredients, and is sure to please.

1. Cut the stems off of the peppers. Slice lengthwise. Remove any seeds that are inside. Set aside.

2. In the bowl of a food processor (or blender), put the chickpeas, yogurt, vinegar, mustard, thyme, and green onions, salt, and cayenne pepper.

3. Pulse 4 or 5 times. The chickpeas should still be a bit chunky.

4. Remove the blade and stir to make sure the mixture is blended well.

5. Stuff each pepper half with about 2 tablespoons of the chickpea mixture.

6. Serve, or store in an airtight container in the refrigerator for up to 3 days.

INGREDIENT TIP: *You can make this recipe dairy free by replacing the yogurt with vegan mayonnaise or mashed silken tofu. You can also vary the beans and spices used depending on your preferences. This snack also makes a healthy appetizer for football season.*

PER SERVING: CALORIES: 34; CARBS: 6G; GLYCEMIC LOAD: 2; FIBER: 2G; SODIUM: 43MG; PROTEIN: 2G; FAT: 0G; SATURATED FAT: 0G

"Cheesy" Popcorn

LOWER CALORIE, INFLAMMATION FIGHTER, DAIRY FREE, GLUTEN FREE

2 tablespoons
  nutritional yeast
⅛ teaspoon ground turmeric
¼ to ½ teaspoon sea salt
¼ teaspoon paprika
  (optional)
¼ teaspoon garlic powder
  (optional)
¼ teaspoon onion powder
  (optional)
⅛ teaspoon cayenne pepper
  (optional)
1 tablespoon coconut oil
  (preferred because of its
  high smoke point)
¼ cup organic corn kernels

SERVES 3 | PREP TIME: 5 MINUTES | COOK TIME: 10 MINUTES

When prepared with the right ingredients, popcorn is low in calories, heart-smart, and surprisingly full of nutrients, making it one of the healthiest snacks you can eat. At a recent American Chemical Society meeting, scientists mentioned that popcorn may contain more polyphenols than some fruits and vegetables. Polyphenols are plant chemicals that help neutralize free radicals in your body. And it is classified as a whole grain. The cheese flavor in this recipe comes from nutritional yeast, a complete protein rich in B vitamins and iron.

1. In a small bowl, add the nutritional yeast, turmeric, salt, and your choice of optional spices. Stir to combine and set aside.

2. In a large lidded saucepan over high heat, add the coconut oil and heat till it melts and is hot.

3. Add 2 to 3 corn kernels and cover the pan with a lid. Shake the pot a little and wait for all 3 to pop. When they do, remove the lid carefully (be careful of the steam), and remove the kernels with a spoon.

4. Add the remaining corn kernels and cover the pan with a lid.

5. Keep the heat on high and shake the pot, holding the lid down so there's no steam escaping.

6. When the corn starts popping, shake the pot every 3 to 5 seconds so the popcorn doesn't burn.

7. When there are 5-second gaps between popping, remove the pan from the heat immediately. Don't try to pop every kernel or you will burn the popcorn.

8. Carefully remove the lid and transfer the popcorn to a big bowl. Sprinkle with the seasoning mix, and toss to coat quickly and well.

9. Serve immediately.

INGREDIENT TIP: *When purchasing the popcorn kernels, consider getting organic popping corn. It isn't much higher in price and the potential health benefits are significant. Organic popping corn will not have the pesticide residues found on conventionally grown corn, and it will not have been genetically engineered.*

PER SERVING: CALORIES: 124; CARBS: 16G; GLYCEMIC LOAD: 8; FIBER: 4G; SODIUM: 391MG; PROTEIN: 5G; FAT: 5G; SATURATED FAT: 4G

Crispy Baked Zucchini Fries

FERTILITY BOOST, LOWER CALORIE, DAIRY FREE, GLUTEN FREE

Olive oil cooking spray
2 medium zucchini, trimmed
2 egg whites
½ cup whole-wheat
    panko bread crumbs
    (see Ingredient Tip)
½ teaspoon dried rosemary
¾ teaspoon garlic powder
¾ teaspoon onion powder
⅛ teaspoon salt
⅛ teaspoon freshly ground
    black pepper

INGREDIENT TIP: *Panko is a type of Japanese bread crumbs traditionally used as a coating for deep-fried foods. The biggest difference between panko and bread crumbs is that panko is made from bread without crusts, so it's tender and the flakes are bigger. You can find plain organic panko at most grocery stores, but if you would rather not use bread, simply replace with almond meal.*

SERVES 2 | PREP TIME: 15 MINUTES | COOK TIME: 20 MINUTES

Veggie-based fried appetizers may sound healthy, but in reality they are a nutritional nightmare, high in unhealthy fats, salt, and calories. This recipe lightens things up to create a satisfying snack or tasty side dish that provides blood sugar–balancing fiber, as much protein as one egg, high levels of the antioxidants vitamins A and C, inflammation-reducing phytochemicals, and fertility-boosting folate.

1. Preheat the oven to 350°F.

2. Spray a large baking sheet with olive oil cooking spray.

3. Cut the zucchini into long spears.

4. Put the zucchini spears in a large bowl. Add the egg whites, and toss gently to coat.

5. In a medium-large bowl, combine the bread crumbs, rosemary, garlic powder, onion powder, salt, and pepper.

6. One at a time, shake zucchini spears to remove excess egg, and lightly coat with bread crumb mixture. Place each spear on the baking sheet, leaving a bit of space between them. Sprinkle with the remaining bread crumbs.

7. Bake for 10 minutes. Carefully flip the spears and bake for an additional 10 minutes until lightly browned and crispy.

8. Let cool for 10 minutes. Serve hot.

PER SERVING: CALORIES: 177; CARBS: 30G; GLYCEMIC LOAD: 19; FIBER: 2G; SODIUM: 376MG; PROTEIN: 9G; FAT: 2G; SATURATED FAT: 0G

Sesame Asparagus

FERTILITY BOOST, LOWER CALORIE, DAIRY FREE, GLUTEN FREE

1 bunch fresh
asparagus, trimmed

1 tablespoon extra-virgin
olive oil

Salt

2 tablespoons black sesame
seeds, lightly toasted
(see Cooking Tip)

Freshly ground black pepper

SERVES 4 | PREP TIME: 5 MINUTES | COOK TIME: 10 MINUTES

This simple recipe uses fresh asparagus, which is a green veggie packed with health benefits. An excellent source of fertility-boosting folate, and the antioxidants vitamin C and E, it is also a good source of chromium, a trace mineral that enhances insulin sensitivity. With a sprinkling of calcium-rich sesame seeds, this light dish makes an excellent side to baked fish, poultry, or tofu.

1. Fill a large saucepan with ½ inch of water and bring it to a boil over medium heat. Add the asparagus and cook until tender crisp, about 5 minutes, being careful not to overcook. Carefully drain the asparagus and rinse it under cold water. Drain well and transfer to a plate.

2. Return the pan to the stove over medium heat, add the olive oil, and swirl it in the bottom of the pan to coat.

3. Add the asparagus to the pan, shaking off any excess water. Season with salt and pepper and toss with the toasted sesame seeds. Cook the asparagus over medium heat until it is warmed through.

4. Serve immediately.

COOKING TIP: *To toast the sesame seeds, toss them in a dry heavy-bottomed skillet over medium heat until they are fragrant. You could also substitute slivered almonds or another of your favorite nuts or seeds. For an omega-3 boost, try using hemp seeds.*

PER SERVING: CALORIES: 81; CARBS: 4G; GLYCEMIC LOAD: 1; FIBER: 2G; SODIUM: 26MG; PROTEIN: 3G; FAT: 7G; SATURATED FAT: 1G

Roasted Vegetables

LOWER CALORIE, INFLAMMATION FIGHTER, DAIRY FREE, GLUTEN FREE

2 tablespoons extra-virgin
olive oil, plus more for
the pan
2 cups bite-size
broccoli florets
2 cups button mushrooms
1 cup diced butternut squash
2 cups chopped green beans
(2-inch pieces)
1 zucchini, quartered
lengthwise and cut
into 2-inch pieces
1 yellow summer
squash, diced
1 red bell pepper, diced
1 red onion, chopped
2 tablespoons
balsamic vinegar
4 garlic cloves, minced
2 teaspoons dried rosemary
1½ teaspoons dried thyme
Salt
Freshly ground black pepper

SERVES 6 | PREP TIME: 15 MINUTES | COOK TIME: 15 MINUTES

If you are a self-proclaimed veggie hater, do yourself a favor and give roasted vegetables a try. Roasting draws out the natural sweetness in vegetables, rewarding you with caramelized, slightly crisp morsels that are much more flavorful than their steamed counterparts. This inflammation-fighting veggie mix is high in vitamins, minerals, and important antioxidants and phytochemicals.

1. Preheat the oven to 425°F.

2. Lightly coat a baking sheet with olive oil.

3. In the prepared pan, spread the broccoli, mushrooms, squash, green beans, zucchini, squash, bell pepper, and red onion in a single layer.

4. Sprinkle the vegetables with the 2 tablespoons olive oil, the balsamic vinegar, garlic, rosemary, and thyme, and season with salt and pepper. Gently toss to combine.

5. Bake for 12 to 15 minutes, or until all the veggies are fork tender.

6. Serve immediately.

FERTILITY BOOST TIP: *For additional folate and vitamins A and C, you could add asparagus, Brussels sprouts, and okra to the mix and sprinkle with shelled sunflower seeds or slivered almonds. Folate is easily destroyed during cooking, especially when moist-heat methods are used, so by using a dry-heat method such as roasting, you can retain more of this important nutrient.*

PER SERVING: CALORIES: 92; CARBS: 11G; GLYCEMIC LOAD: 4; FIBER: 3G; SODIUM: 33MG; PROTEIN: 3G; FAT: 5G; SATURATED FAT: 1G

Shredded Brussels Sprouts with Nuts and Berries

FERTILITY BOOST, LOWER CALORIE, INFLAMMATION FIGHTER, DAIRY FREE, GLUTEN FREE

1 pound Brussels sprouts, trimmed
2 teaspoons extra-virgin olive oil, divided
½ red onion, diced
⅓ cup shelled pistachios, roughly chopped
½ cup fresh cranberries
1 tablespoon hemp seeds
Salt
½ teaspoon freshly ground black pepper

INFLAMMATION FIGHTER TIP: *One way to reduce inflammation in your body is to shift your balance of dietary fats to emphasize omega-3 fats over omega-6 fats. Nuts and seeds contain high amounts of omega-3 fats and can be used as a garnish for most recipes. Just keep an eye on portion size because they are rather dense in calories.*

SERVES 8 | PREP TIME: 15 MINUTES | COOK TIME: 10 MINUTES

Not only are pistachios a source of many essential vitamins and minerals, healthy fats, protein, and fiber, but they also provide an array of phytochemicals. Studies indicate that pistachios may help maintain healthy blood glucose levels as well as lower the blood sugar response when eaten with carbohydrates like rice and pasta. A 1-ounce serving of pistachios equals 49 nuts, which is more nuts per serving than any other snack nut. Enjoy this tasty side dish with grilled fish, poultry, or tofu.

1. Cut each Brussels sprout in half through the stem, and cut into thin slices.

2. Heat 1 teaspoon of the olive oil in a large skillet over medium heat. Add the onion and cook, stirring occasionally, until it begins to soften, 4 to 5 minutes.

3. Add the remaining 1 teaspoon olive oil to the skillet, and then add the Brussels sprouts. Cook, stirring occasionally, until the Brussels sprouts are almost tender but still bright green.

4. Stir in the pistachios, cranberries, and hemp seeds, and season with salt and add the pepper.

5. Serve immediately.

PER SERVING: CALORIES: 113; CARBS: 12G; GLYCEMIC LOAD: 5; FIBER: 3G; SODIUM: 27MG; PROTEIN: 4G; FAT: 7G; SATURATED FAT: 1G

Roasted Brussels Sprouts, Red Onion, and Apple

FERTILITY BOOST, LOWER CALORIE, INFLAMMATION FIGHTER, DAIRY FREE, GLUTEN FREE

Olive oil cooking spray
1 pound Brussels sprouts, fairly equal in size, trimmed
2 medium red onions, cut into 2-inch chunks
2 medium Yellow Delicious apples, cored and cut into 2-inch chunks
2 tablespoons extra-virgin olive oil
1 tablespoon minced garlic
1 teaspoon mustard powder
1 teaspoon smoked paprika
1 teaspoon salt
¼ teaspoon freshly ground black pepper

INFLAMMATION FIGHTER TIP: *Apples are an excellent food to work into your eating plan, due to their low glycemic load and high amounts of phyto-nutrients, antioxidants, and heart-healthy soluble fiber. Including apples in your diet may reduce your risk of devel-oping cancer, hypertension, heart disease, and diabetes. Add chopped apples to both sweet and savory dishes for a nutritional boost.*

SERVES 4 | PREP TIME: 10 MINUTES | COOK TIME: 15 MINUTES

Oven roasting brings out the sweet flavor of the Brussels sprouts and keeps them crisp while toning down their characteristic strong flavor. Full of fertility-boosting folate and fiber, this is an excellent side dish to cooked beans, fish, poultry, or meats. You will need skewers; soak bamboo or wooden skewers in water for 30 minutes before cooking to avoid burning.

1. Preheat the oven to 400°F.

2. Lightly coat a baking sheet with olive oil cooking spray.

3. Put the Brussels sprouts in a large, microwave-safe mixing bowl and heat them on high for 3 minutes.

4. Remove the Brussels sprouts from the microwave and add the onions, apples, olive oil, garlic, mustard, paprika, and salt, and toss to combine.

5. On each skewer, alternate the Brussels sprouts with red onion and apple in any order you prefer, leaving about ½ inch between each food item.

6. Place the skewers on the prepared baking sheet. Roast for 10 to 15 minutes until the Brussels sprouts, onions, and apples are crisp on the outside and tender on the inside.

7. Add the black pepper and serve hot.

PER SERVING: CALORIES: 178; CARBS: 28G; GLYCEMIC LOAD: 8; FIBER: 7G; SODIUM: 613MG; PROTEIN: 5G; FAT: 7G; SATURATED FAT: 1G

Garlic-Lemon Swiss Chard and Butter Beans

FERTILITY BOOST, LOWER CALORIE, INFLAMMATION FIGHTER, DAIRY FREE, GLUTEN FREE

1 large bunch Swiss chard, washed and shaken dry

2 teaspoons extra-virgin olive oil, plus more if needed

2 teaspoons minced garlic

1 (15-ounce) can butter beans, drained and rinsed (or an equal amount cooked fresh or frozen lima beans)

2 tablespoons freshly squeezed lemon juice, plus more if needed

Salt

Freshly ground black pepper

COOKING TIP: *If you have the time and they are in season, the taste of fresh lima beans is well worth the effort. You'll need 2 pounds of fresh beans for this recipe. Shell and wash them thoroughly, then place them in a saucepan over low heat with 2 cups water and a dash of salt. Cover and simmer until tender, about 30 minutes.*

SERVES 2 TO 3 | PREP TIME: 5 MINUTES | COOK TIME: 10 MINUTES

Low-glycemic-index butter beans have a delicate flavor that complements a wide variety of dishes, and in this recipe they are paired with sturdy Swiss chard. Nutritionally, each serving is packed with protein and fiber, providing steady energy and ample amounts of heart-healthy and fertility-boosting folate and magnesium.

1. Slice each chard leaf lengthwise on both sides of the stem. Discard the stems (or save them for another use). Stack the chard leaves and cut them crosswise into ¾-inch-thick strips.

2. Heat the olive oil in a large pot over medium heat, swirling the pan to coat. When the oil begins to shimmer, add the garlic and stir for about 30 seconds until fragrant and light brown.

3. Stir in the chard, cover the pot, reduce the heat to medium low, and cook for 5 minutes or until the chard has wilted.

4. Remove the lid from the pot and gently stir in the beans and lemon juice; season with salt and pepper. Cook for 4 to 5 minutes, stirring occasionally. Add a drizzle of olive oil if the beans start to dry out.

5. Taste and add more lemon juice, salt, and/or pepper if desired. Serve hot.

PER SERVING: CALORIES: 295; CARBS: 46G; GLYCEMIC LOAD: 19; FIBER: 13G; SODIUM: 290MG; PROTEIN: 18G; FAT: 6G; SATURATED FAT: 1G

Portobello Eggs with Sun-Dried Tomatoes

FERTILITY BOOST, LOWER CALORIE, DAIRY FREE, GLUTEN FREE

2 portobello mushroom caps

Olive oil cooking spray

2 tablespoons finely chopped sun-dried tomatoes (not packed in oil)

2 eggs

⅛ teaspoon garlic powder

Salt

Freshly ground black pepper

¼ cup chopped fresh basil, for garnish

SERVES 2 | PREP TIME: 5 MINUTES | COOK TIME: 15 MINUTES

Easy and nutritious, this dish may become your new go-to favorite for a vegetarian snack or side dish. It requires only four ingredients (plus salt and pepper). In this recipe, meaty, high-fiber, vitamin D–rich portobello mushrooms are stuffed with egg and topped with sun-dried tomatoes to create a delicious flavor combination. Tomatoes are an excellent source of vitamins C, A, and E, and the phytochemical lycopene, which can reduce cancer risk. Serve over a big salad, with sautéed greens, with soup, or enjoy as a snack.

1. Preheat the oven to 400°F. Line a baking sheet with aluminum foil.

2. Remove the stems from the mushroom caps and scrape out the gills with a spoon.

3. Coat both sides of the mushroom caps with olive oil cooking spray, or lightly brush them with olive oil, and set them upside-down on the prepared baking sheet.

4. Sprinkle the sun-dried tomatoes into the mushroom caps, dividing them equally.

5. Crack an egg into each mushroom cap, attempting to get the yolk to sit in the cavity where you removed the stem so it stays in place.

6. Carefully transfer the baking sheet to the oven, and bake for 15 minutes or until the egg whites are opaque and the eggs have set.

7. Remove the baking sheet from the oven and season the mushrooms with the garlic powder, salt, and pepper.

8. Sprinkle with the basil and serve hot.

COOKING TIP: *Try to choose portobello mushrooms that are about 3 ounces each, with a wide lip to hold in the yolks. If the egg yolks break or run slightly off the mushrooms during cooking, just reduce the cooking time by a few minutes to avoid overcooking the yolk.*

PER SERVING: CALORIES: 124; CARBS: 8G; GLYCEMIC LOAD: 4; FIBER: 3G; SODIUM: 208MG; PROTEIN: 12G; FAT: 6G; SATURATED FAT: 2G

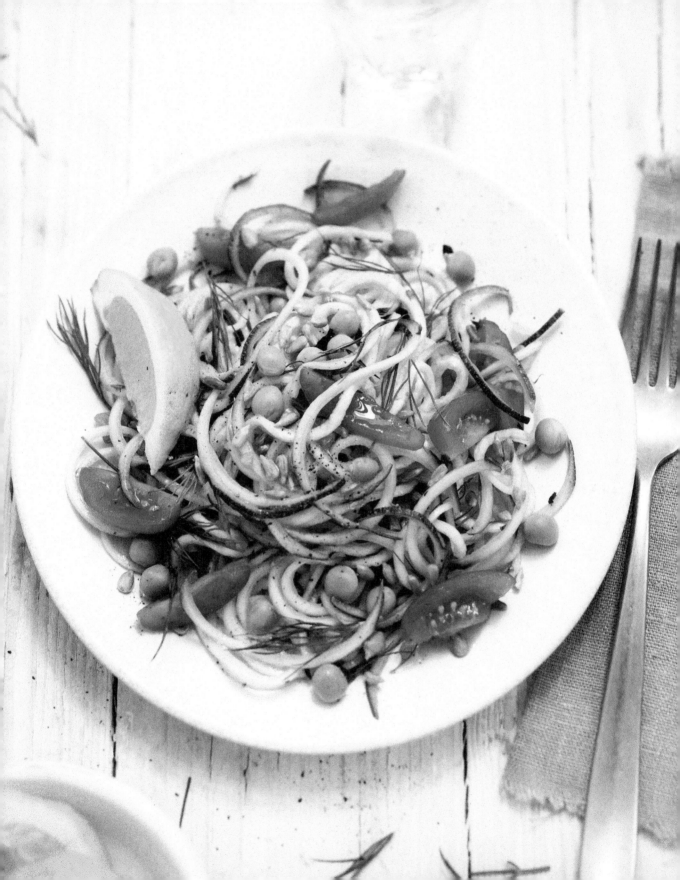

6

Vegetarian and Vegan Entrées

One-Pan Asparagus Eggs

FERTILITY BOOST, LOWER CALORIE, INFLAMMATION FIGHTER, DAIRY FREE, GLUTEN FREE

Olive oil cooking spray
1 pound asparagus, trimmed
1 pint cherry tomatoes
1 tablespoon extra-virgin
    olive oil
2 garlic cloves, minced
¼ cup chopped fresh
    basil leaves
Salt
Freshly ground black pepper
4 eggs

INFLAMMATION
FIGHTER TIP: *Cooking
with herbs and spices is
an excellent way to add
valuable antioxidants and
inflammation-fighting phytochemicals to your diet. Basil is
one of the most potent anti-
inflammatory herbs, along with
ginger, rosemary, and turmeric,
which would all work well in
this recipe.*

SERVES 4 | PREP TIME: 5 MINUTES | COOK TIME: 20 MINUTES

*This baked egg dish is a simple, elegant, no-fuss meal that
makes a satisfying and nutritious dinner. Eggs are an all-
natural source of high-quality protein; 13 essential vitamins
and minerals, including vitamins A, D, and E; and carotenoids lutein and zeaxanthin. Though eggs were once tied
to high cholesterol and resulting heart issues, the 2015–2020
Dietary Guidelines for Americans reports that cholesterol is
not a nutrient of concern for overconsumption, so you can
freely enjoy eggs without fear of their cholesterol content.*

1. Preheat the oven to 400°F. Coat a baking sheet with
olive oil cooking spray.

2. Arrange the asparagus and cherry tomatoes in an
even layer on the prepared baking sheet. Drizzle the
olive oil over the vegetables. Sprinkle with the garlic and
basil, and season with salt and pepper.

3. Roast until the asparagus is nearly tender and the
tomatoes are wrinkled, 10 to 12 minutes.

4. Crack the eggs on top of the vegetables, and season
each with salt and pepper.

5. Bake until the egg whites are set and the yolks are
still soft, 7 to 8 minutes.

6. Remove the baking sheet from the oven and divide
the asparagus, tomatoes, and eggs among 4 plates;
serve hot.

PER SERVING: CALORIES: 133; CARBS: 7G; GLYCEMIC LOAD: 3; FIBER: 3G;
SODIUM: 99MG; PROTEIN: 9G; FAT: 9G; SATURATED FAT: 2G

Almond-Crusted Tofu

INFLAMMATION FIGHTER, DAIRY FREE, GLUTEN FREE

2 egg whites
1 cup almond meal
½ teaspoon paprika
½ teaspoon garlic powder
½ teaspoon salt
½ teaspoon freshly ground
    black pepper
1 (15- or 16-ounce) block
    organic extra-firm tofu,
    cut into 12 squares,
    drained and patted dry

INGREDIENT TIP: *You can make this recipe vegan by replacing the egg whites with 3 tablespoons of powdered egg replacer mixed with 8 tablespoons of water. Alternatively, you could also make flaxseed eggs: Whisk together 3 tablespoons of flaxseed meal and 8 tablespoons of water. Refrigerate for 10 minutes to thicken.*

SERVES 4 | PREP TIME: 30 MINUTES | COOK TIME: 25 MINUTES

Tofu is an excellent food to incorporate into an anti-inflammatory diet, yet many people shy away because they don't know how to cook it. If you haven't tried tofu yet, consider the health benefits. Tofu is one of the few plant-based proteins that contain all essential amino acids, are loaded with calcium and iron, and are low in calories—a perfect healthy alternative to meat. This recipe is delicious and easy to prepare, and the tofu is crispy from baking, not frying. Serve it over a salad, brown rice and vegetables, or a baked sweet potato.

1. Preheat the oven to 375°F. Line a baking sheet with parchment paper.

2. In a small shallow bowl, whisk the egg whites.

3. In another small shallow bowl, whisk together the almond meal, paprika, garlic powder, salt, and pepper.

4. Dip each square of tofu into the egg whites, letting the excess fall back into the dish.

5. Press all sides of each tofu square into the almond meal mixture to coat. Place the coated tofu squares on the prepared baking sheet, cover, and refrigerate for at least 20 minutes to set the crust.

6. Bake for approximately 20 to 25 minutes until golden and crispy.

7. Serve immediately.

PER SERVING: CALORIES: 104; CARBS: 3G; GLYCEMIC LOAD: 2; FIBER: 0G; SODIUM: 389MG; PROTEIN: 11G; FAT: 5G; SATURATED FAT: 0G

Cauliflower Fried Rice

LOWER CALORIE, INFLAMMATION FIGHTER, DAIRY FREE, GLUTEN FREE

24 ounces (about 5 cups)
   cauliflower florets
2 tablespoons Bragg's
   liquid aminos
1 tablespoon toasted
   sesame oil
1 tablespoon peeled and
   minced fresh ginger
¼ teaspoon freshly ground
   white pepper
2 teaspoons
   plus 1 tablespoon
   olive oil, divided
2 eggs, beaten
2 garlic cloves, minced
1 medium white onion, diced
½ cup bite-size
   broccoli florets
1 red bell pepper, chopped
2 medium carrots, peeled
   and grated
1 cup snow peas
2 green onions, thinly sliced
   (white and light
   green parts)
1 teaspoon sesame seeds

SERVES 4 | PREP TIME: 10 MINUTES | COOK TIME: 10 MINUTES

This recipe is a healthy twist on traditional fried rice, which is typically loaded with unhealthy fats, MSG, high-glycemic carbs, and sodium. Riced cauliflower is used in place of refined white rice in this dish, and Bragg's liquid aminos replaces traditional soy sauce. With several servings of vegetables in each portion, this protein- and fiber-rich dish will give you slow-burning, fertility-boosting energy.

1. To make the cauliflower rice, put the cauliflower in the bowl of a food processor (or blender) and pulse until it resembles rice, 2 to 3 minutes; set aside.

2. In a small bowl, whisk together the aminos, sesame oil, ginger, and white pepper; set aside.

3. Heat 2 teaspoons of the olive oil in a medium skillet over low heat. Swirl the oil in the pan so it coats the bottom. Add the eggs and cook, 2 to 3 minutes per side, flipping only once. Let cool, then chop into small pieces and set aside on a plate.

4. Heat the remaining tablespoon of olive oil in a large skillet or wok over medium-high heat. Add the garlic and onion and cook, stirring often, until the onion has become translucent, 3 to 4 minutes. Stir in the broccoli, bell pepper, carrots, and snow peas. Cook, stirring constantly, until the vegetables are crisp tender, 3 to 4 minutes.

5. Stir in the cauliflower, chopped eggs, green onions, and aminos mixture. Cook, stirring constantly, until everything is heated through and the cauliflower is tender, 3 to 4 minutes.

6. Serve hot, garnished with the sesame seeds.

INFLAMMATION FIGHTER TIP: *For an added crunch and boost of antioxidants, add in a few sliced water chestnuts. Water chestnuts are a good source of phenolics, a type of flavonoid that exerts powerful anti-inflammatory effects in the body.*

PER SERVING: CALORIES: 195; CARBS: 21G; GLYCEMIC LOAD: 9; FIBER: 8G; SODIUM: 618MG; PROTEIN: 10G; FAT: 9G; SATURATED FAT: 2G

Mini Crustless Quiches

FERTILITY BOOSTING, LOWER CALORIE, DAIRY FREE, GLUTEN FREE

Olive oil cooking spray
1 tablespoon olive oil
½ cup finely chopped
    white onion
½ cup finely chopped
    mushrooms
½ cup finely chopped
    green bell pepper
¼ cup finely chopped
    tomatoes
1 cup frozen and thawed
    spinach or kale
6 eggs
½ teaspoon dried thyme
¼ cup nutritional yeast
    (optional)
Salt
Freshly ground black pepper

MAKES 12 SMALL OR 6 LARGER QUICHES
PREP TIME: 10 MINUTES | COOK TIME: 15 MINUTES

Mini quiches are great options to prepare in advance for those busy weeknights when you need to put a healthy dinner on the table fast. Full of high-quality protein and nutrient-rich veggies, these quiches can be made with whatever vegetables you have on hand. Serve with a salad and low-glycemic grain like quinoa for a balanced, satisfying meal. They are also portable and kid-friendly and can serve double duty as a grab-and-go snack or breakfast.

1. Preheat the oven to 350°F.

2. Coat the cups of a standard 12-cup muffin tin with olive oil cooking spray.

3. Heat the olive oil in a large skillet over medium heat. Add the onion, mushrooms, bell pepper, tomatoes, and spinach and sauté until the vegetables have softened, about 5 minutes. Remove the skillet from the heat.

4. Whisk the eggs in a medium bowl. Add the thyme and nutritional yeast (if using), and season with salt and pepper. Stir in the sautéed veggies.

5. Fill each of the prepared muffin cups ¾ of the way to the top with the egg mixture (this recipe makes 12 low or 6 taller quiches).

6. Bake for 10 to 15 minutes for low quiches or 15 to 20 minutes for taller quiches. They are done when the egg mixture has set and is firm to the touch.

7. Remove the quiches from the oven and let them cool slightly.

8. Serve warm or wrap the quiches in plastic and refrigerate for up to 3 days.

INFLAMMATION FIGHTER TIP: *While optional, nutritional yeast adds more than a nondairy cheese type of taste. This nutritional powerhouse contains high levels of B vitamins, folic acid, selenium, zinc, and protein. It is low in fat, is gluten free, and contains no added sugars or preservatives.*

PER SERVING: CALORIES: 51; CARBS: 1G; GLYCEMIC LOAD: 1; FIBER: 0G; SODIUM: 38MG; PROTEIN: 3G; FAT: 4G; SATURATED FAT: 1G

Grilled Cauliflower Steaks with Mango and Black Bean Salsa

FERTILITY BOOST, LOWER CALORIE, DAIRY FREE, GLUTEN FREE

1 large head cauliflower

2 tablespoons extra-virgin olive oil

Salt

Freshly ground black pepper

1½ cups cherry tomatoes

2 cups chopped fresh mango

1 (15-ounce) can black beans, drained and rinsed

¼ cup chopped fresh cilantro

2 green onions, thinly sliced (white and light green parts)

Juice of 2 limes

½ teaspoon ground cumin

1 teaspoon chili powder

½ teaspoon paprika

1 avocado, sliced

LOWER CALORIE TIP: *While this recipe is already low in calories, you could easily omit the fruit from the recipe and replace it with a low-calorie vegetable like chopped red bell pepper, red onion, chopped celery, or tomatillos. You could also add grilled tofu for additional protein.*

SERVES 4 | PREP TIME: 10 MINUTES | COOK TIME: 8 MINUTES

This vegan entrée is full of blood sugar–stabilizing protein and fiber, and rich in fertility-boosting antioxidants, vitamins, and minerals. Top each serving of this delicious, high-protein dish with sliced avocado for additional fiber and healthy fats.

1. Remove the outer leaves and extended stem from the head of cauliflower. Working from the center, cut four horizontal, 1-inch-thick steaks. Steaks can only be made with the florets attached to the core stem. Florets that detach from the core can be cooked on the side or reserved for another use.

2. Heat a grill or grill pan to medium-high heat. Brush each side of the cauliflower steaks with some of the olive oil, and sprinkle with salt and pepper. Grill each side for 3 to 4 minutes until lightly charred.

3. For the fresh salsa, cut the cherry tomatoes into quarters and put them in a medium bowl.

4. Add the mango, beans, cilantro, green onions, lime juice, cumin, chili powder, and paprika, and season lightly with salt and pepper. Stir to combine.

5. To serve, place a cauliflower steak on each of 4 plates, and spoon mounds of salsa on top.

6. Garnish with avocado slices and serve.

PER SERVING: CALORIES: 374; CARBS: 56G; GLYCEMIC LOAD: 19; FIBER: 19G; SODIUM: 97MG; PROTEIN: 15G; FAT: 13G; SATURATED FAT: 2G

Tofu Kale Scramble

INFLAMMATION FIGHTER, DAIRY FREE, GLUTEN FREE

1 (15-ounce) package
   non-GMO extra-firm tofu
2 teaspoons olive oil
¼ cup nutritional yeast
1 teaspoon ground turmeric
1 teaspoon paprika
1 teaspoon garlic powder
2 cups stemmed and
   chopped kale
½ cup halved cherry
   tomatoes
¼ cup chopped green
   onions (white and light
   green parts)
1 large avocado, diced
Salt
Freshly ground black pepper

LOWER CALORIE TIP: *While avocadoes are rich in healthy fats, soluble fiber, vitamins, and minerals, they are also an energy-dense food, meaning that it is important to watch portion sizes. To lower the calorie count of this recipe, simply reduce the amount of diced avocado to 1 or 2 tablespoons per serving.*

SERVES 4 | PREP TIME: 5 MINUTES | COOK TIME: 15 MINUTES

Including adequate protein at each meal is essential for keeping you feeling full, maintaining blood sugar levels, and decreasing your cravings for less healthy foods. This easy tofu scramble is high in complete plant-based protein, includes the nutritional powerhouse kale, and gets healthy fats from chunks of avocado. With the anti-inflammatory spice turmeric added for color, how could this dish be any healthier?

1. Drain the liquid from the tofu container, put the tofu block on a plate, and cut it into long strips. Stack the strips on the plate, separating them with paper towels. Place something with a bit of weight (like a heavy dish) on top of the stacked tofu, and set it aside for a few minutes to drain.

2. When the tofu has drained, heat the olive oil in a large skillet over medium heat. Add the tofu strips and use a spatula to break them up into smaller pieces.

3. In a small bowl, stir together the nutritional yeast, turmeric, paprika, and garlic powder. Sprinkle this mixture over the tofu and stir well, so each piece of tofu is seasoned.

4. Add the kale, tomatoes, and green onions to the skillet and cook, tossing frequently, until the kale is tender, about 10 minutes.

5. Stir in the avocado and season with salt and pepper.

6. Serve hot.

PER SERVING: CALORIES: 207; CARBS: 14G; GLYCEMIC LOAD: 5; FIBER: 7G; SODIUM: 113MG; PROTEIN: 14G; FAT: 13G; SATURATED FAT: 2G

Navy Bean and Quinoa Loaf

FERTILITY BOOST, LOWER CALORIE, INFLAMMATION FIGHTER, DAIRY FREE, GLUTEN FREE

Olive oil cooking spray
3 tablespoons chia seeds
½ cup warm water
1 tablespoon olive oil
1 medium onion, chopped
4 garlic cloves, minced
2 celery stalks, chopped
8 ounces button
    mushrooms, sliced
1 (15-ounce) can navy beans,
    drained and rinsed
¾ cup old-fashioned
    rolled oats
2 tablespoons Bragg's
    liquid aminos
2 cups cooked quinoa
10 sun-dried tomatoes
    packed in oil, drained
    and chopped
1 tablespoon minced
    fresh thyme
½ teaspoon salt
½ teaspoon freshly ground
    black pepper

SERVES 8 | PREP TIME: 15 MINUTES, PLUS 15 MINUTES TO CHILL
COOK TIME: 70 MINUTES

Taking time on the weekends to prepare one or two entrées is a great way to save time, and cooking in bulk means leftovers can be used for lunches or frozen for later. This quinoa and bean loaf recipe is very flexible—you can use any type of bean or grain and vary the vegetables and spices to your liking. Navy beans are featured here because of their high amounts of folate, which supports fertility; magnesium and potassium, which help protect the heart; and tryptophan, an essential amino acid that you need to stay emotionally calm. Soaking the chia seeds in warm water creates a gel-like mixture that can serves as a vegan substitute for egg whites.

1. Preheat the oven to 350°F. Lightly coat an 8-by-4-inch loaf pan with olive oil cooking spray.

2. In a small bowl, mix the chia seeds with the warm water and stir well. Refrigerate for at least 15 minutes, until the mixture forms a gel or a "chia egg."

3. Heat the olive oil in a medium skillet over medium heat. Add the onion, garlic, celery, and mushrooms, and sauté for 4 to 5 minutes.

4. In a food processor (or blender), combine the beans, oats, and aminos; pulse until almost smooth.

5. In a large bowl, combine the quinoa, bean mixture, onion mixture, sun-dried tomatoes, chia egg, thyme, salt, and pepper.

6. Transfer the mixture to the prepared loaf pan, pressing it gently to fill the pan and mounding it slightly in the middle.

7. Bake until golden brown and firm, about 1 hour.

8. Remove the loaf from the oven and set it aside to rest for 10 minutes before slicing and serving hot.

COOKING TIP: *Serve any leftover slices of this loaf on toasted sprouted bread, or make lettuce wraps with a touch of spicy mustard. You can also cook the loaf mixture in mini-loaf pans for easier portion control.*

PER SERVING: CALORIES: 253; CARBS: 40G; GLYCEMIC LOAD: 16; FIBER: 11G; SODIUM: 421MG; PROTEIN: 15G; FAT: 6G; SATURATED FAT: 1G

Kung Pao Tempeh

LOWER CALORIE, INFLAMMATION FIGHTER, DAIRY FREE, GLUTEN FREE

8 ounces organic tempeh

½ cup tamari sauce

1 teaspoon peeled and grated fresh ginger

2 teaspoons agave nectar or honey

1 garlic cloves, minced

1 tablespoon rice vinegar

1 teaspoon toasted sesame oil

1 tablespoon olive oil

1 teaspoon arrowroot powder or cornstarch

3 green onions, sliced (white and light green parts), and some for garnish (optional)

1 cup snow peas

1 medium red bell pepper, chopped

1 medium green bell pepper, chopped

1 medium yellow summer squash, chopped

1 teaspoon crushed red pepper flakes

¼ cup unsalted peanuts

SERVES 4 | PREP TIME: 20 MINUTES, PLUS 10 MINUTES TO MARINATE | COOK TIME: 10 MINUTES

Don't be intimidated by the list of ingredients; the taste of this recipe is well worth it. Tempeh, a type of fermented soy, has a meaty, chewy texture that works well as a meat substitute. This very low-GI food contains high amounts of natural probiotics, which keep your intestinal tract healthy, as well as protein, vitamins, minerals, and inflammation-reducing phytochemicals. This delicious vegan dish has all the flavor of traditional Chinese Kung Pao, but without the meat and less-healthy ingredients.

1. Set a small steamer basket in a small saucepan over medium-high heat. Add about 1 inch of water and bring it to a boil.

2. Cut the tempeh into 4 slices and transfer to the steamer basket. Cover and steam for about 10 minutes.

3. Meanwhile, in a medium bowl, whisk together the tamari, ginger, agave nectar, garlic, rice vinegar, and sesame oil.

4. Remove the tempeh from the steamer, cut it into bite-size chunks, and add it to the tamari mixture. Marinate the tempeh for at least 10 minutes at room temperature.

5. Heat the olive oil in a large skillet or wok over medium heat. Add the tempeh and sauté gently until it turns golden brown, about 5 minutes.

6. Whisk the arrowroot into the remaining marinade and add it to the pan, stirring the sauce. Add the green onions, snow peas, red bell pepper, green bell pepper, summer squash, red pepper flakes, and peanuts. Cook until vegetables are tender, about 5 minutes, sautéing quickly but gently so the tempeh doesn't crumble.

7. Remove the pan from the heat and serve immediately. Ganish with the remaining chopped green onion (if using).

INGREDIENT TIP: *The trick to cooking with tempeh is to steam it first so it will absorb the most flavor. Cut one brick into 4 squares, steam for 10 minutes, then marinate for 10 minutes, then sauté or bake and include in any recipe. Or just eat it plain.*

PER SERVING: CALORIES: 281; CARBS: 22G; GLYCEMIC LOAD: 11; FIBER: 3G; SODIUM: 2023MG; PROTEIN: 18G; FAT: 15G; SATURATED FAT: 3G

Zucchini Pasta with Tomatoes and Peas

LOWER CALORIE, DAIRY FREE, GLUTEN FREE

3 medium zucchini
½ tablespoon extra-virgin olive oil
3 garlic cloves, minced
4 Roma tomatoes, quartered, with their juices
1 cup frozen green peas
Salt
Freshly ground black pepper
2 tablespoons sunflower seeds
1 bunch fresh dill, for garnish
1 lemon, cut into wedges for serving

INFLAMMATION FIGHTER TIP: *For additional inflammation-fighting power, add 1 sliced red onion to the skillet with the garlic. The onion will increase the amount of inflammation-fighting phytochemicals and add 15 percent of the recommended daily value of the antioxidant vitamin C.*

SERVES 4 | PREP TIME: 10 MINUTES | COOK TIME: 10 MINUTES

One of the tricks to managing your weight without feeling hungry is to fill your plate with high-volume, nutrient-dense foods. A great way to do this is to spiralize veggies and use them as a replacement for traditional pasta. A spiral vegetable slicer is easy to use and costs less than a couple of coffee drinks. If you don't have one, peel the zucchini into super-thin strips, rotating the zucchini after each strip. This recipe is powered by plant protein from green peas, a vegetable with unique phytonutrients, providing antioxidant and anti-inflammatory benefits. With healthy fats and vitamin E from sunflower seeds, this fresh-tasting and nutritious dish is both filling and satisfying.

1. Feed the zucchini through a vegetable spiralizer or mandoline, or cut it into thin strips with a vegetable peeler.

2. Heat the olive oil in a large skillet over medium heat. Add the garlic and sauté until the garlic is fragrant, 2 to 3 minutes. Add the tomatoes, their juices, and the peas, and cook until the peas are thawed.

3. Add the zucchini pasta to the vegetable mixture. Toss to combine, and cook until the zucchini is heated through, about 3 minutes. Season with salt and pepper to taste.

4. Serve hot, garnished with the sunflower seeds, fresh dill, and lemon wedges.

PER SERVING: CALORIES: 80; CARBS: 9G; GLYCEMIC LOAD: 3; FIBER: 3G; SODIUM: 64MG; PROTEIN: 3G; FAT: 4G; SATURATED FAT: 0G

Vegan "Crab" Cakes

FERTILITY BOOST, LOWER CALORIE, INFLAMMATION FIGHTER, DAIRY FREE, GLUTEN FREE

FOR THE SAUCE

¼ cup mashed avocado

1 tablespoon tahini
(sesame paste)

1 tablespoon extra-virgin
olive oil

1 tablespoon freshly
squeezed lemon juice

Salt

FOR THE "CRAB" CAKES

1 (14-ounce) can hearts of
palm, drained and diced

¼ cup mashed avocado

¼ cup diced red bell pepper

¼ cup diced red onion

2 garlic cloves, minced

2 teaspoons Old Bay
seasoning

½ teaspoon ground ginger

1 cup cooked quinoa

Salt

Freshly ground black pepper

¼ cup gluten-free flour
(chickpea, quinoa,
or almond)

2 tablespoons olive oil

LOWER CALORIE TIP: *While
each crab cake is already low
in calories, you could use a
dry heat cooking method and
bake the cakes, which would
lower the calorie count further
by eliminating the use of the
olive oil.*

SERVES 6 | PREP TIME: 20 MINUTES, PLUS 15 MINUTES
TO FREEZE | COOK TIME: 8 MINUTES

*This recipe title may sound like an oxymoron, but thanks to
one fantastic ingredient, known as hearts of palm, it is possible to make patties that taste just like crabcakes! Hearts of
palm are very low in calories yet high in fiber, fertility-boosting
folate, vitamin C, and blood pressure–regulating potassium
and magnesium. Once chopped or shredded, hearts of palm
perfectly mimic that crab-like texture, and the addition of
quinoa brings protein to the mix.*

TO MAKE THE SAUCE

In a blender, combine the avocado, tahini, olive oil, and
lemon juice, and season with salt. Blend until smooth,
then pour the sauce into a small bowl for serving.

TO MAKE THE "CRAB" CAKES

1. In a medium bowl, combine the hearts of palm, avocado, red bell pepper, onion, garlic, Old Bay, ginger, and
cooked quinoa, and season with salt and pepper. Mix
well. Add the gluten-free flour and mix until combined.

2. Form the mixture into 6 rounded patties. Freeze for
15 to 20 minutes (freezing helps them stay together
when cooked).

3. In a medium skillet over medium heat, warm the
olive oil. Panfry the patties until they are browned on
each side, about 4 minutes per side.

4. Serve immediately, passing the sauce at the table.

PER SERVING: CALORIES: 199; CARBS: 20G; GLYCEMIC LOAD: 7; FIBER: 9G;
SODIUM: 243MG; PROTEIN: 5G; FAT: 12G; SATURATED FAT: 2G

Spinach, Sweet Potato, and Lentil Dal

LOWER CALORIE, INFLAMMATION FIGHTER, DAIRY FREE, GLUTEN FREE

1 tablespoon olive oil

1 medium white onion, diced

2 garlic cloves, chopped

1-inch piece fresh ginger, peeled and minced

1 medium sweet potato, diced

1 cup chopped tomatoes

1 small red or yellow bell pepper, chopped

4 cups low-sodium vegetable broth

1 cup dried red lentils

2 tablespoons medium to hot curry powder (or use your own spice mix; see Inflammation Fighter Tip)

2 cups chopped baby spinach leaves

SERVES 4 | PREP TIME: 10 MINUTES | COOK TIME: 25 MINUTES

Dal, which can also be spelled Dahl, Dhal, or Daal, is a simple Indian lentil soup or stew, usually made with ghee or clarified butter. Here, though, it is made with olive oil, an ingredient with healthier types of fats. High in satiating protein and fiber, this recipe is also rich in the beta-carotene from the sweet potato; folate, iron, and B vitamins from the lentils; and vitamins A and C and phytochemicals from the spinach. If you want to make your own spice mix for this recipe, see the Inflammation Fighter Tip below. Serve the dal with a dollop of Greek yogurt or over brown rice.

1. Heat the olive oil in a large skillet over medium heat until it begins to shimmer. Add the onion, garlic, and ginger, and sauté until the onion is translucent, about 5 minutes.

2. Add the sweet potato, tomatoes, bell pepper, broth, and lentils. Cover the pan and simmer for 10 minutes.

3. Add the curry powder (or use your own spice mix) and stir well. Cover and simmer for 10 minutes, until the dal has thickened and the sweet potato is soft.

4. Remove the pan from the heat. Add the spinach, and gently stir until it wilts.

5. Serve immediately.

INFLAMMATION FIGHTER TIP: *Using premade curry powder is a time saver, but putting together your own spice mix assures that the spices are fresh and allows you to tailor it to your taste preferences. To make your own, mix together 1 teaspoon ground cumin, 1 teaspoon ground turmeric, 1 teaspoon garam masala, 1 teaspoon cayenne pepper, 1 teaspoon ground coriander, ½ teaspoon ground cinnamon, and ½ teaspoon ground ginger. Use the same proportion of curry spices as in the recipe. Store the rest of the spice mix in a jar in a cool, dark cupboard. Turmeric is one of the most powerful anti-inflammatory spices there is, so consider increasing the amount used, depending on your health needs.*

PER SERVING: CALORIES: 266; CARBS: 45G; GLYCEMIC LOAD: 19; FIBER: 8G; SODIUM: 578MG; PROTEIN: 14G; FAT: 5G; SATURATED FAT: 1G

Baked Broccoli and Bean Burgers

LOWER CALORIE, INFLAMMATION FIGHTER, DAIRY FREE, GLUTEN FREE

⅓ cup uncooked quinoa
1 cup water
1½ cups broccoli florets
2 teaspoons olive oil
½ cup chopped green onions (white and light green parts)
½ cup chopped red onion
2 garlic cloves, minced
2 teaspoons ground cumin
1 (15-ounce) can chickpeas (garbanzo beans), drained and rinsed
¼ cup almond meal or almond flour
1 tablespoon tahini (sesame paste)

SERVES 4 | PREP TIME: 30 MINUTES | COOK TIME: 75 MINUTES

Homemade veggie burgers are a great way to sneak vegetables into your diet or the diet of the picky eaters in your household. This recipe features the cruciferous powerhouse, broccoli, one of the most popular veggies in the United States. The fiber in broccoli can help keep cholesterol in check, and the vitamin A and K content can promote vitamin D absorption in the body. High in vitamin C, folate, and flavonoids, broccoli stands out among vegetables for its antioxidant and anti-inflammatory benefits. Top the burgers with your favorite accompaniments, such as tomato slices, lettuce, pickles, mustard, avocado, and Sriracha sauce.

1. Preheat the oven to 400°F. Line a baking sheet with aluminum foil.

2. Put the quinoa in a fine-mesh sieve and rinse it under cool water, rubbing to remove the bitter outer coating. Drain well.

3. Bring 1 cup of water to a boil in a small saucepan over high heat. Add the quinoa, reduce the heat to medium, and cook for 15 minutes. Drain the quinoa and set it aside.

4. Meanwhile, set a small steamer basket in a small lidded pot and pour in 1 inch of water. Bring the water to a boil over high heat. Place the broccoli in the steamer basket, cover, reduce the heat to medium, and steam for 5 to 7 minutes.

5. Heat the olive oil in a medium skillet over medium heat. Add the green onion, red onion, and garlic, and sauté, stirring occasionally, for 3 to 5 minutes until the onion softens. Remove the skillet from the heat and stir in the cumin.

6. In a food processor (or blender), combine the quinoa, broccoli, onion mixture, chickpeas, almond meal, and tahini; pulse until combined.

7. Form the mixture into 4 patties and place them on the prepared baking sheet.

8. Bake for 50 minutes, turning the patties halfway through. They should be browned and slightly firm to the touch.

9. Remove the patties from the oven and serve hot.

INGREDIENT TIP: *You can use any type of bean or grain in this recipe and add in additional chopped veggies for more health benefits. You could also vary the type of binder you use—maybe substitute chickpea flour or panko for the almond meal.*

PER SERVING: CALORIES: 299; CARBS: 44G; GLYCEMIC LOAD: 18; FIBER: 11G; SODIUM: 27MG; PROTEIN: 14G; FAT: 9G; SATURATED FAT: 1G

Cauliflower Crust Pizza

FERTILITY BOOST, LOWER CALORIE, INFLAMMATION FIGHTER, DAIRY FREE, GLUTEN FREE

2½ tablespoons flaxseed meal or chia seeds (or use 1 whole egg)

¼ cup warm water

½ medium head cauliflower, chopped into florets

⅓ cup chickpea flour (or substitute coconut, almond, or oat flour)

1 garlic clove, minced

½ teaspoon dried oregano

½ teaspoon dried basil

½ teaspoon salt

½ teaspoon freshly ground black pepper

2 tablespoons nutritional yeast (optional)

¼ cup chopped fresh basil leaves (optional)

SERVES 2 TO 4 | PREP TIME: 20 MINUTES, PLUS 30 MINUTES CHILLING TIME | COOK TIME: 30 MINUTES

Grated cauliflower does more than make a great rice substitute, it also works as a unique and tasty replacement for traditional high-carb, high-glycemic pizza dough. Another bonus? A ½-cup serving of cauliflower provides over 70 percent of the recommended daily allowance for the antioxidant vitamin C. Plus, cauliflower is a very good source of vitamin K, folate, and B vitamins, has a low GI, and is rich in inflammation-reducing phytonutrients. This is so good you will forget it's healthy! The nutritional yeast offers a cheesy flavor and is a complete protein, rich in B vitamins and iron.

1. In a small bowl, whisk together the flaxseed meal and water, and refrigerate for at least 30 minutes or until thickened.

2. Preheat the oven to 450°F. Line a baking sheet with aluminum foil.

3. Set a small steamer basket in a small saucepan, add 1 inch of water, cover, and bring to a boil over medium heat.

4. Add cauliflower florets to the steamer, cover, and steam until they are soft and falling apart, 3 to 5 minutes. Drain completely.

5. Put the cauliflower in a clean dishcloth or a large piece of cheesecloth, and holding it over a bowl, squeeze out the excess water from the cauliflower. You want it as dry as possible, so at least ⅔ cup water should come out.

6. Discard the cauliflower liquid; the squeezed cauliflower will resemble a firm purée.

7. Place the squeezed cauliflower in a medium bowl and add the thickened flaxseed mixture. Mash and stir well.

8. In a small bowl, mix together the chickpea flour, garlic, oregano, dried basil, salt, black pepper, nutritional yeast (if using), and fresh basil (if using). Mix well. Add the flour mixture to the cauliflower mixture and mix well.

9. Form the dough into a ball and place it on the prepared pan. Pat the dough into a circle and spread it out to a ¼- to ½-inch thickness. You don't want it too thin, because the moisture will cause it to crack.

10. Bake for about 20 minutes, until the top is golden brown and firm to the touch. You can flip it halfway through baking, if you like.

11. Remove the crust from the oven, and reduce the oven temperature to 400°F.

12. Top the pizza crust with your favorite toppings, then return it to the oven and bake for another 8 to 10 minutes or until the toppings have heated. Serve hot.

COOKING TIP: *To save time, buy pre-riced or grated cauliflower. Grated cauliflower is easy to find in the produce section of most grocery stores, and large natural food markets usually carry it in the frozen vegetable section.*

PER SERVING: CALORIES: 89; CARBS: 8G; GLYCEMIC LOAD: 4; FIBER: 4G; SODIUM: 660MG; PROTEIN: 7G; FAT: 4G; SATURATED FAT: 1G

Split Pea Falafel

FERTILITY BOOST, LOWER CALORIE, INFLAMMATION FIGHTER, DAIRY FREE, GLUTEN FREE

½ cup dried green split peas

2 cups water

⅓ cup chopped red onion

4 garlic cloves

½ cup packed fresh
  flat-leaf parsley

½ teaspoon salt

1 teaspoon ground cumin

1 teaspoon ground coriander

½ teaspoon freshly ground
  black pepper

2 teaspoons olive oil, plus
  more for your hands and
  for brushing

1 to 2 tablespoons
  chickpea flour

2 tablespoons sesame seeds
  (optional)

2 tablespoons tahini
  (sesame paste)
  (optional)

SERVES 4 | PREP TIME: 15 MINUTES | COOK TIME: 50 MINUTES

Falafel is a traditional Middle Eastern dish of spiced, mashed chickpeas that are formed into small balls and then deep-fried. This unique twist on the dish replaces chickpeas with the higher protein split pea and lowers the calories by baking instead of frying. Split peas are very high in fiber and can help stabilize blood sugar by supplying steady energy. Rich in B-vitamins, a serving of dried peas contains over 300 percent of the recommended daily amount of molybdenum, a trace mineral that contributes to antioxidant protection. Enjoy on top of a salad, with a dollop of tahini, or stuffed into a sprouted grain pita pocket.

1. Preheat the oven to 400°F.

2. In a colander, pick over and wash the split peas. Drain.

3. In a medium saucepan over medium-high heat, combine the split peas and the water. Bring the water to a boil and cook until the peas are tender, 18 to 20 minutes. Drain the peas and let them cool slightly.

4. Put the peas in a food processor (or blender). Add the onion, garlic, parsley, salt, cumin, coriander, pepper, and olive oil; pulse to make a coarse mixture. Transfer to a medium bowl. Add the chickpea flour and stir, as needed, to make the dough less sticky.

5. Line a baking sheet with parchment paper.

6. Grease your hands with some olive oil and shape the dough into 1½-inch balls. Place the balls on the prepared pan. Brush more olive oil on top. Sprinkle with sesame seeds (if using).

7. Bake for 30 minutes or until the falafel is golden and crisp on the outside.

8. Remove the baking sheet from the oven and serve the falafel immediately, with tahini (if using).

COOKING TIP: *Any type of hummus would make a tasty topper for this dish. Or you could whip up your own tahini sauce by whisking together ⅓ cup tahini, 2 tablespoons freshly squeezed lemon juice, 3 to 4 tablespoons water, and some salt and freshly ground white pepper.*

PER SERVING: CALORIES: 127; CARBS: 19G; GLYCEMIC LOAD: 7; FIBER: 7G; SODIUM: 301MG; PROTEIN: 7G; FAT: 3G; SATURATED FAT: 0G

Braised Coconut Spinach and Chickpeas

INFLAMMATION FIGHTER, DAIRY FREE, GLUTEN FREE

2 teaspoons olive oil

1 small yellow onion, diced

1 medium red bell
  pepper, chopped

4 garlic cloves, minced

1 tablespoon peeled and
  grated fresh ginger

½ cup sun-dried
  tomatoes, chopped

Zest and juice of
  1 large lemon

1 (15-ounce) can chickpeas
  (garbanzo beans), drained
  and rinsed

10 gently packed cups
  baby spinach

1 (14-ounce) can light
  coconut milk

½ teaspoon salt

1 teaspoon ground ginger

2 large cooked sweet
  potatoes cut in half,
  for serving (optional)

½ cup chopped cilantro
  leaves, for garnish

SERVES 4 | PREP TIME: 10 MINUTES | COOK TIME: 25 MINUTES

This spicy, tangy dish of braised greens and chickpeas is slow-cooked with garlic, ginger, and onion in a creamy coconut milk sauce. Dairy free and vegan, you'll get several servings of nutrient-rich vegetables high in vitamins A, C, and folate along with blood sugar–stabilizing protein from fiber-rich chickpeas. Vegan comfort food at its best, this stew is thick enough to eat with a fork but is designed to be served over cooked sweet potatoes or grains.

1. Heat the olive oil in a large Dutch oven over medium-high heat. Add the onion and bell pepper and sauté for about 5 minutes, or until the onion is beginning to brown.

2. Add the garlic, ginger, sun-dried tomatoes, and lemon zest. Sauté for 3 minutes.

3. Add the chickpeas and sauté for 2 to 3 minutes, or until the chickpeas begin to turn golden and are coated with the onion and garlic mixture.

4. Add the spinach, a handful at a time, and stir. (This will take about 5 minutes. Stir in a handful and wait for it to wilt down and make room in the pot before adding the next handful. Repeat until all the spinach is wilted.) Pour in the coconut milk, salt, ground ginger, and lemon juice. Bring to a simmer, then turn down the heat to low and cook for 10 minutes, or until the chickpeas are warmed through. Taste and add more salt if necessary.

5. Serve over the sweet potatoes (if using) and garnish with the fresh cilantro.

INFLAMMATION FIGHTER TIP: *Sweet potatoes are a superfood on so many levels. They have a low glycemic index; they are easy to find, store, and cook; and 1 cup has over 65 percent of the daily recommendation for vitamin C and 700 percent of the daily recommendation for vitamin A. High in fiber and free radical–fighting phytochemicals, this vegetable is delicious, and you can feel good about including it in your meal plan.*

PER SERVING: CALORIES: 405; CARBS: 41G; GLYCEMIC LOAD: 16; FIBER: 11G; SODIUM: 516MG; PROTEIN: 14G; FAT: 23G; SATURATED FAT: 17G

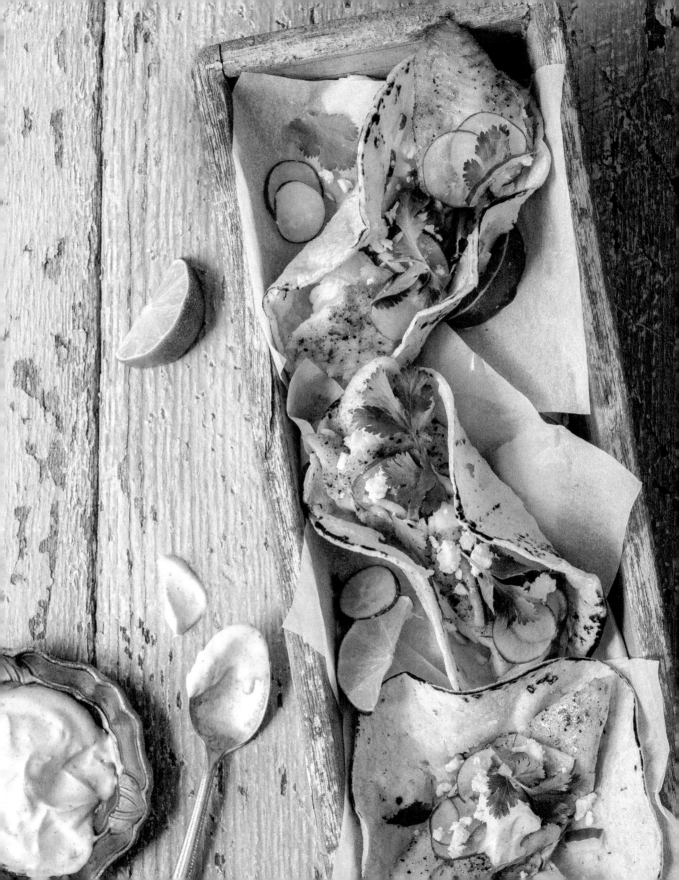

7

Fish and Seafood

Salmon with Mushrooms and Brussels Sprouts

INFLAMMATION FIGHTER, DAIRY FREE, GLUTEN FREE

FOR THE VEGETABLES

Olive oil cooking spray

1 pound Brussels sprouts,
  end trimmed, sliced in half

1 cup shiitake mushrooms

1 tablespoon olive oil

½ teaspoon salt

¼ teaspoon freshly ground
  black pepper

FOR THE SALMON

1-pound wild-caught salmon
  fillet, cut into 4 portions

2 teaspoons olive oil

3 garlic cloves, minced

1 tablespoon dried oregano

½ teaspoon salt

½ teaspoon freshly ground
  black pepper

¼ cup chopped fresh chives,
  for garnish

SERVES 4 | PREP TIME: 10 MINUTES | COOK TIME: 30 MINUTES

The Dietary Guidelines for Americans, *the American Heart Association, and the American Diabetes Association all recommend eating at least two servings of fatty fish each week for optimal health and disease risk reduction. Salmon is one of the best sources of these essential, inflammation-reducing, heart-healthy fats, and is readily accessible and easy to prepare. In this one-pan recipe, salmon is oven-roasted with folate-rich Brussels sprouts and vitamin D–rich mushroom for a meal that is simple enough for a weeknight dinner yet sophisticated enough for company.*

TO MAKE THE VEGETABLES

1. Preheat the oven to 450°F.

2. Lightly coat a baking sheet with olive oil cooking spray.

3. In a large mixing bowl, combine the Brussels sprouts, mushrooms, olive oil, salt, and pepper, and toss until well mixed. Transfer to the prepared pan, and spread in a single layer. Bake for 15 minutes, stirring once or twice.

TO MAKE THE SALMON

1. Meanwhile, drizzle salmon portions with the olive oil, and put some of the minced garlic on top of the 4 portions. Sprinkle with the oregano, salt, and pepper.

2. Remove the baking sheet from oven. Move the vegetables over, making 4 empty spots for the salmon fillets. Place the salmon fillets on the pan. Bake the salmon for 10 to 12 minutes until it is cooked through and flakes when pricked with a fork.

3. Let stand for 2 minutes. Serve hot, garnished with the chives.

FERTILITY BOOST TIP: *You can enhance the fertility-boosting power of this recipe by roasting cauliflower florets, which are a good source of choline, as well as asparagus, another great source of folate. Filling up on vegetables is an excellent way to add valuable nutrients and blood sugar–stabilizing fiber to your diet while increasing the overall satiety of the meal.*

PER SERVING: CALORIES: 313; CARBS: 13G; GLYCEMIC LOAD: 5; FIBER: 5G; SODIUM: 373MG; PROTEIN: 27G; FAT: 18G; SATURATED FAT: 4G

Grilled Salmon with Pomegranate, Mint, and Pine Nut Couscous

GLUTEN FREE, DAIRY FREE, INFLAMMATION FIGHTER

4 (6-ounce) wild caught
  salmon filets
3 tablespoons extra virgin
  olive oil
½ teaspoon salt
½ teaspoon pepper

FOR THE COUSCOUS
1 cup dried whole-wheat
  couscous
1 cup water
2 tablespoons fresh
  lemon juice
1 tablespoon olive oil
½ cup pomegranate seeds
½ cup chopped celery
¼ cup pine nuts
¼ cup fresh mint, chopped
  plus more for garnish
¼ cup fresh parsley, chopped
  plus more for garnish
1 lemon, cut into wedges
  for garnish
salt and black pepper to taste

INGREDIENT TIP: *When purchasing salmon, one thing you don't have to worry about is genetically modified salmon hitting the market anytime soon—the FDA banned the sale, at least for now. The best advice is to inquire about farming practices, contaminants, and nutritional content as omega-3 content may vary.*

SERVES 4 | PREP TIME: 10 MINUTES | COOK TIME: 15 MINUTES

Wild-caught salmon has a reputation for being heart healthy, due to its extraordinarily high omega-3 fatty acid content. Eating 2–3 servings of fatty fish like salmon per week has been shown to reduce inflammation and lower triglycerides. This delicious recipe packs a potent anti-inflammatory punch.

1. Preheat grill or grill pan. Prepare the salmon by brushing on olive oil. Sprinkle with salt and pepper.

2. Grill the salmon over direct heat on the first side, about 6 to 7 minutes. Turn fish and cook on the second side, about 5 to 6 minutes. Fish should be opaque or reach an internal temperature of 140 degrees.

3. While the salmon cooks, prepare the couscous by bringing the water to boil in a medium pot over high heat. When the water boils, remove pot from the heat, mix in the couscous, cover, and let sit for 5 minutes.

4. Fluff the couscous with a fork.

5. In a large mixing bowl, whisk together olive oil, lemon juice, pomegranate seeds, celery, pine nuts, fresh mint, fresh parsley, and salt and pepper to taste. Add couscous and gently incorporate dressing and couscous with a fork.

6. To serve, divide the couscous between 4 serving plates and top each with a piece of salmon.

PER SERVING: CALORIES: 662; CARBS: 40G; GLYCEMIC LOAD: 24; FIBER: 4G; PROTEIN: 41G; SODIUM: 386MG; FAT: 37G

Salmon, Apple, and Avocado Wrap

INFLAMMATION FIGHTER, DAIRY FREE, GLUTEN FREE

1 pound wild-caught
  salmon fillet
½ teaspoon salt
¼ teaspoon freshly ground
  black pepper
2 limes
1 medium tomato, diced
1 large avocado, diced
1 medium apple, diced
1 tablespoon chopped
  fresh mint
1 tablespoon olive oil
1 head romaine lettuce

INFLAMMATION FIGHTER TIP: *You could increase the anti-inflammatory power of this meal by adding 2 minced garlic cloves to the fresh salsa. Garlic contains a compound called allicin, which has been shown to lower blood triglycerides and total cholesterol (NCCIH, 2016). The anti-inflammatory compounds can also reduce total low-level bodily inflammation.*

SERVES 4 | PREP TIME: 10 MINUTES | COOK TIME: 15 MINUTES

These flavorful wraps are as nutritious as they are delicious. Inflammation-fighting salmon is baked and topped with a fresh salsa made from apple and avocado, then wrapped in lettuce leaves. Apples are an excellent source of heart-healthy fiber, important antioxidants, and flavonoid phytochemicals that may help reduce the risk for heart disease, diabetes, hypertension, and cancer.

1. Preheat the oven to 425°F.

2. Line a baking sheet with aluminum foil.

3. Place the salmon fillet in the prepared pan. Season with the salt and pepper. Slice one lime and spread the slices evenly on top of the salmon fillet. Bake for 15 minutes, or until the salmon is cooked through. It will look opaque and will flake when pierced with a fork.

4. Meanwhile, in a medium bowl, combine the tomato, avocado, and apple. Set aside.

5. In a small bowl, combine the chopped mint, olive oil, and the juice of one freshly squeezed lime. Whisk to combine.

6. Wash and dry the lettuce leaves.

7. Flake the salmon into the apple-avocado mixture. Add the mint dressing and mix well.

8. Scoop ¼ of the mixture into the center of each piece of lettuce. Roll up to eat.

PER SERVING: CALORIES: 377; CARBS: 19G; GLYCEMIC LOAD: 5; FIBER: 9G; SODIUM: 359MG; PROTEIN: 26G; FAT: 23G; SATURATED FAT: 6G

Fish Tacos

LOWER CALORIE, GLUTEN FREE

FOR THE TACOS

1 pound firm white fish
   (such as tilapia, cod,
   or catfish)
2 medium limes, halved
1 garlic clove, minced
1 teaspoon ground cumin
¼ teaspoon chili powder
½ teaspoon oregano
4 teaspoons olive oil,
   divided, plus more
   for the grill
Salt
Freshly ground black pepper
½ small head of red cabbage,
   cored and thinly sliced
½ cup radishes, thinly sliced
½ red onion, thinly sliced
½ cup chopped fresh cilantro
8 (6-inch) organic corn
   tortillas
crumbled white cheddar
   cheese (optional for
   topping)

FOR THE WHITE SAUCE

½ cup nonfat plain
   Greek yogurt
1 teaspoon sriracha hot sauce
½ teaspoon crushed oregano
½ teaspoon ground cumin
½ teaspoon dill
Freshly ground black pepper
   to taste
Fresh lime juice to taste

SERVES 4 | PREP TIME: 20 MINUTES, PLUS 15 MINUTES
TO MARINATE | COOK TIME: 11 MINUTES

While restaurant-style battered and fried fish tacos are deli-cious, they are high in calories and fat and not particularly healthy. With this recipe you can satisfy your cravings while nourishing your body with high-quality protein and a serving or two of vegetables. Corn tortillas are lower on the glycemic index than flour tortillas, making them a good choice for load-ing up with grilled fish in this speedy lunch or dinner.

TO MAKE THE TACOS

1. Place the fish pieces in a baking dish and squeeze a lime half over it. Over the fish, sprinkle the garlic, cumin, chili powder, oregano, and 3 teaspoons of the olive oil. Season with salt and pepper. Turn the fish in the mari-nade until evenly coated. Refrigerate and let marinate at least 15 minutes.

2. In a medium-sized bowl, combine the radishes, onion, and cilantro and squeeze a lime half over it. Drizzle with the remaining 1 teaspoon olive oil, and season with salt and pepper. Toss to combine, and set aside.

TO MAKE THE WHITE SAUCE

In a small bowl, combine the yogurt, sriracha, oregano, cumin, dill, pepper, and lime juice, and mix until com-bined. Set aside.

TO ASSEMBLE THE TACOS

1. In a medium skillet over medium-high heat, warm the tortillas one at a time, flipping to warm both sides, about 5 minutes total. Wrap the warm tortillas in a clean dishcloth and set them aside while you prepare the fish.

2. Brush the grates of a grill pan or outdoor grill with oil and heat over medium-high heat until hot. Remove the fish from the marinade and place on the grill.

3. Cook the fish without moving it until the underside has grill marks and is white and opaque on the bottom, about 3 minutes. Flip and grill the other side until white and opaque, 2 to 3 minutes more. Transfer the fish to a plate.

4. Break off some of the cooked fish, place it in a warm tortilla, and top it with the radish mixture, some crumbled white cheddar cheese (if using), and a squeeze of lime. Drizzle with white sauce.

LOWER CALORIE TIP: *You could make this recipe lower in calories and higher in vitamins, minerals, and antioxidants by leaving out the white sauce and replacing the corn tortilla with a sturdy green for wrapping. Collard greens make a great choice, and you can simply use them raw or blanch the leaves to make them more pliable and easy to work with.*

PER SERVING: CALORIES: 290; CARBS: 28G; GLYCEMIC LOAD: 14; FIBER: 3G; SODIUM: 146MG; PROTEIN: 27G; FAT: 8G; SATURATED FAT: 2G

Thai Halibut and Brown Rice Lettuce Wraps

DAIRY FREE, GLUTEN FREE

4 (1-inch-thick, 4-ounce) fresh halibut fillets

¼ teaspoon salt

¼ teaspoon freshly ground black pepper

1 tablespoon sesame oil

2 tablespoons rice vinegar

1 tablespoon freshly squeezed lime juice

1 teaspoon honey

½ teaspoon crushed red pepper flakes

1 cup cooked brown rice

1 medium red bell pepper, thinly sliced

1 cup snow peas, trimmed and thinly sliced diagonally

¼ cup thinly sliced green onions (white and light green parts)

¼ cup chopped fresh cilantro

8 to 12 leaves butter lettuce (Boston or Bibb) or romaine lettuce

1 tablespoon cashews, coarsely chopped

2 tablespoons chia seeds (optional)

LOWER CALORIE TIP: *Lower the calories further by replacing the rice with grated cauliflower, zucchini, or carrot ribbons. This keeps the fiber and vitamin C content high.*

SERVES 4 | PREP TIME: 10 MINUTES | COOK TIME: 20 MINUTES

Lettuce wraps are easy to make, tasty, and will keep you feeling full and energized without excess calories from bread or tortillas. Halibut has a sweet, delicate flavor with a snow-white flesh, contains few bones, and is a good source of high-quality protein, as well as omega-3 fatty acids, selenium, magnesium, and potassium, all of which are important for heart health. Mixed with B vitamins– and fiber-rich brown rice, these light and delicious wraps are a handheld treat.

1. Sprinkle the halibut with the salt and pepper.

2. Heat the sesame oil in a large skillet over medium heat. Add the fish and cook for 8 to 12 minutes, or until the fish flakes easily when tested with a fork, turning to brown both sides.

3. In a small bowl, combine the rice vinegar, lime juice, honey, and red pepper flakes.

4. Place one cooked halibut steak on each of 4 dinner plates. Portion out the rice, red bell pepper, snow peas, green onions, cilantro, and 2 to 3 lettuce leaves onto the 4 plates.

5. To eat, spoon some of the fish, rice, vegetables, and cilantro into one of the lettuce leaves. Drizzle with the rice vinegar mixture and sprinkle with the cashews and chia seeds (if using). Roll up to eat.

PER SERVING: CALORIES: 265; CARBS: 18G; GLYCEMIC LOAD: 8; FIBER: 2G; SODIUM: 216MG; PROTEIN: 26G; FAT: 9G; SATURATED FAT: 1G

Halibut with Lentils and Mustard Sauce

INFLAMMATION FIGHTER, DAIRY FREE, GLUTEN FREE

2 tablespoons olive oil, divided

1 medium red onion, chopped

2 garlic cloves, chopped

1 cup Brussels sprouts, halved

2½ cups low-sodium vegetable broth, plus ¼ cup

1¼ cup dried green lentils, rinsed

¾ teaspoon salt, divided

¾ teaspoon freshly ground black pepper, divided

4 (6-ounce) pieces halibut fillet

¼ cup Dijon mustard

1 tablespoon chopped fresh tarragon

FERTILITY BOOST TIP: *You could boost the choline content in this recipe by steaming riced cauliflower and serving the fish and lentil dish over the "rice." Most women don't get enough choline, yet it is a nutrient with the potential to reduce harmful gene effects that may result in birth defects.*

SERVES 4 | PREP TIME: 10 MINUTES | COOK TIME: 35 MINUTES

This protein-rich dish combines lentils with the low-calorie, delicate taste of halibut, creating a meal that will provide long-lasting energy without any spikes in blood sugar. The addition of tarragon brings high levels of free radical–neutralizing antioxidants, as well as good amounts of vitamins A, C, and B_6, magnesium, iron, zinc, and calcium.

1. Heat 1 tablespoon of the olive oil in a large skillet over medium heat. Add the onion and cook, stirring occasionally, until soft, 5 to 6 minutes.

2. Add the garlic and Brussels sprouts and cook, stirring, for 1 minute.

3. Add 2½ cups of the broth and the lentils and simmer, covered, until the lentils are tender, 20 to 25 minutes. Season with ½ teaspoon of the salt and ½ teaspoon of the pepper.

4. Meanwhile, heat the remaining tablespoon of oil in a medium skillet over medium-high heat. Season the fish with the remaining ¼ teaspoon salt and the remaining ¼ teaspoon pepper. Cook until opaque throughout, 3 to 5 minutes per side.

5. In a small bowl, whisk together the mustard, the remaining ¼ cup broth, and the tarragon. Divide the lentil mixture and the fish among 4 plates and drizzle with the mustard-tarragon sauce.

PER SERVING: CALORIES: 492; CARBS: 43G; GLYCEMIC LOAD: 20; FIBER: 8G; SODIUM: 646MG; PROTEIN: 52G; FAT: 13G; SATURATED FAT: 2G

Cod with Sugar Snap Peas

LOWER CALORIE, DAIRY FREE, GLUTEN FREE

1 tablespoon freshly
   squeezed lime juice
1 teaspoon peeled and grated
   fresh ginger
2 tablespoons olive oil,
   divided
¾ teaspoon salt, divided
½ teaspoon freshly ground
   black pepper, divided
4 cups sugar snap peas,
   strings removed
1 cup button mushrooms
1 medium carrot, peeled
   and grated
1 tablespoon sesame seeds
4 (6-ounce) pieces cod fillet
1 lime cut into 4 wedges

INFLAMMATION

FIGHTER TIP: *You can easily boost the inflammation power of any recipe by simply adding onions. Onions contain chromium, which assists in regulating blood sugar, and their phytochemicals and vitamin C content help improve immunity. In terms of the best onion to choose, researchers found that shallots and Western yellow onions have the highest phenolic and flavonoid content.*

SERVES 4 | PREP TIME: 10 MINUTES | COOK TIME: 10 MINUTES

This simple, nutritious, and delicious meal of fish and veggies takes only minutes to prepare and is perfect for a summer meal. Mild-flavored cod is available throughout the year, but any white fish could be used in this recipe. Cod has a very low GI, and because it is a cold water fish, it is also high in omega-3 fatty acids, which are beneficial for reducing the risks of diabetes and cardiovascular disease. The delicate flavor of the cod works well with the mushrooms, and the sugar snap peas add a welcome crunch.

1. In a large bowl, combine the lime juice, ginger, 1 tablespoon of the oil, ¼ teaspoon salt, and ¼ teaspoon pepper.

2. Add the snap peas, mushrooms, carrot, and sesame seeds, and toss to coat.

3. Heat the remaining tablespoon of oil in a large nonstick skillet over medium-high heat.

4. Season the cod with ½ teaspoon salt and ¼ teaspoon pepper.

5. Add the fish to the skillet and cook until opaque throughout, 3 to 5 minutes per side.

6. Serve with the vegetable salad and lime wedges.

PER SERVING: CALORIES: 269; CARBS: 10G; GLYCEMIC LOAD: 4; FIBER: 4G; SODIUM: 543MG; PROTEIN: 34G; FAT: 10G; SATURATED FAT: 1G

Asian-Style Haddock in Parchment

LOWER CALORIE, DAIRY FREE, GLUTEN FREE

4 (6-ounce) haddock fillets

4 baby bok choy, ends
    trimmed

1 cup small oyster
    mushrooms

1 red bell pepper, thinly sliced

1 cup finely shredded green
    or savoy cabbage

½ teaspoon freshly ground
    black pepper

3 green onions, thinly sliced
    on the diagonal (white and
    light green parts)

2 tablespoons Bragg's
    liquid aminos

1½ teaspoon rice vinegar

1½ teaspoon sesame oil

2 teaspoons peeled and
    grated fresh ginger

FERTILITY BOOST TIP:

*You could vary the vege-
tables in this recipe for more
fertility-boosting folate and
vitamin D. Consider using a
mix of folate-rich bok choy,
asparagus spears, several
different types of mushrooms
(enoki, shiitake, oyster, and
chanterelles), and some finely
shredded spinach.*

SERVES 4 | PREP TIME: 10 MINUTES | COOK TIME: 15 MINUTES

*Cooking fish in parchment paper is easy and healthy. This
steaming technique yields moist, tender results, and a little
oil goes a long way, adding lots of flavor to this otherwise
low-fat cooking technique. In this recipe, low-calorie haddock
is steamed with a mix of Asian-style vegetables and given an
antioxidant boost by the addition of grated fresh ginger.*

1. Heat the oven to 400°F.

2. Tear off eight 15-inch squares of parchment paper
(you can substitute aluminum foil) and arrange two
squares each on two baking sheets.

3. Divide the bok choy, mushrooms, bell pepper, and
cabbage evenly among the four parchment squares.
Place a haddock fillet on top of each, sprinkle with the
black pepper, and top with the green onions.

4. In a small bowl, whisk together the aminos,
vinegar, oil, and ginger. Spoon the mixture evenly over
the haddock.

5. Top each fillet with one of the remaining squares
of parchment, and fold the edges over several times
to seal.

6. Bake for 15 minutes or until the fish is easily flaked
with a fork.

7. Transfer each packet to a plate. Serve with a knife to
split the packet open.

PER SERVING: CALORIES: 194; CARBS: 6G; GLYCEMIC LOAD: 2; FIBER: 2G;
SODIUM: 636MG; PROTEIN: 34G; FAT: 3G; SATURATED FAT: 0G

Tilapia and Vegetable Packets

LOWER CALORIE, DAIRY FREE, GLUTEN FREE

1 cup cherry or grape
tomatoes, quartered

1 cup diced summer squash
(like zucchini,
yellow squash, or
pattypan squash)

1 cup diced eggplant

1 cup thinly sliced red onion

12 green beans, trimmed and
cut into 1-inch pieces

2 tablespoons freshly
squeezed lemon juice

1 tablespoon extra-virgin
olive oil

Small bunch fresh dill,
chopped

½ teaspoon salt, divided

1 teaspoon freshly ground
black pepper, divided

Olive oil cooking spray

1 pound tilapia fillets, cut
into 4 equal portions

SERVES 4 | PREP TIME: 30 MINUTES
COOK TIME: 5 TO 10 MINUTES

This foolproof recipe can be prepared on a grill or in the oven, and is a perfect combination of tastes with the bright flavors of fresh dill and lemon seasoning the vegetables and fish. Dill is an exceptional source of anti-inflammatory phytochemicals and a good source of vitamins A and C, with trace amounts of folate, iron, and manganese. The healthy omega-3 fats and significant amount of high-quality protein in tilapia promote steady blood sugar levels for lasting energy.

1. Preheat a grill or grill pan to medium heat.

2. In a large bowl, combine the tomatoes, squash, eggplant, onion, green beans, lemon juice, olive oil, dill, ¼ teaspoon salt, and ¼ teaspoon pepper.

3. To make a packet, lay two 20-inch-long sheets of foil on top of each other (the double layers will help protect the contents from burning). Generously coat the top sheet of foil with olive oil cooking spray. Place one portion of tilapia in the center of the foil. Sprinkle with some of the remaining ¼ teaspoon salt and ¼ teaspoon pepper, then top with about ¾ cup of the vegetable mixture. Bring the short ends of the foil together, leaving enough room in the packet for steam to gather and cook the food. Fold the foil over and pinch to seal. Pinch the seams together along the sides. Make sure all the seams are tightly sealed to prevent steam from escaping. Repeat to make the other 3 packets.

4. Grill the packets until the fish is cooked through and is easily flaked with a fork, and the vegetables are just tender, about 5 minutes.

5. To serve, carefully open both ends of the packets and allow the steam to escape. Use a spatula to slide the contents onto plates.

COOKING TIP: *For the oven variation, preheat the oven to 425°F. Place the green beans in a microwaveable bowl with 1 tablespoon water. Microwave on high until the beans are just a little tender, about 30 seconds. Drain and add to the other vegetables. Assemble the packets. Bake the packets directly on an oven rack until the tilapia is cooked through and the vegetables are just tender, about 20 minutes.*

PER SERVING: CALORIES: 174; CARBS: 8G; GLYCEMIC LOAD: 3; FIBER: 3G; SODIUM: 355MG; PROTEIN: 24G; FAT: 5G; SATURATED FAT: 1G

Mediterranean Shrimp Kabobs

LOWER CALORIE, INFLAMMATION FIGHTER, DAIRY FREE, GLUTEN FREE

1 pound peeled and deveined
   jumbo shrimp
1 cup cherry tomatoes
½ medium red onion,
   cut in ½-inch cubes
12 canned small
   artichoke hearts
1 medium zucchini, cut
   into rounds
1 green bell pepper,
   cut in 1-inch cubes
12 large pitted black olives
¼ cup extra-virgin olive oil
¼ cup freshly squeezed
   lemon juice
1 teaspoon dried oregano
1 teaspoon dried basil
1 teaspoon garlic powder
¼ teaspoon salt

INFLAMMATION
FIGHTER TIP: *Olives are
another very low-GI food, rich
in dozens of health-protective
nutrients. Technically a fruit,
olives provide heart-healthy
monounsaturated fats and
phytonutrients, and are a good
source of iron, fiber, copper,
and vitamin E. Add them to
salads or cooked grains, or
serve them in a small bowl on
the dinner table for your family
to enjoy with meals.*

SERVES 4 | PREP TIME: 20 MINUTES, PLUS 15 MINUTES
TO MARINATE | COOK TIME: 8 MINUTES

*Shrimp are a very low-calorie, very low-GI food, rich in
high-quality protein and heart-healthy omega-3 fats. Shrimp
feature at least three unique antioxidants, including the
carotenoid astaxanthin, and the minerals selenium and
copper, all of which can reduce the risk for developing type 2
diabetes and cardiovascular disease. Soak 4 bamboo skewers
in water for 30 minutes before using, to prevent burning.*

1. Assemble the skewers by threading the shrimp,
tomatoes, onion, artichoke hearts, zucchini, bell pepper,
and olives on four 12- to 14-inch skewers in whatever
sequence you prefer.

2. In a small bowl, whisk together the olive oil, lemon
juice, oregano, basil, garlic powder, and salt.

3. Place the skewers in a shallow baking dish and pour
half of the marinade over them; cover and refrigerate
for 15 minutes.

4. When you're ready to cook, heat a grill or grill pan
to medium heat. Cook the skewers for 3 minutes on
each side until the shrimp are opaque and cooked
through and the vegetables are soft. Discard the
shrimp marinade.

5. Brush the remaining unused marinade on the
skewers and cook for 2 more minutes.

6. Remove the skewers from the grill and place them on
a serving platter; serve hot.

PER SERVING: CALORIES: 290; CARBS: 11G; GLYCEMIC LOAD: 4; FIBER: 5G;
SODIUM: 457MG; PROTEIN: 25G; FAT: 17G; SATURATED FAT: 2G

Scallops with Sugar Snap Peas

LOWER CALORIE, INFLAMMATION FIGHTER, DAIRY FREE, GLUTEN FREE

3 teaspoons olive oil, divided

12 ounces sugar snap peas, trimmed and sliced diagonally

1 medium red bell pepper, sliced

¼ teaspoon salt, divided

¼ teaspoon freshly ground black pepper, divided

2 large shallots, sliced

1½ pounds large sea scallops

4 lemon wedges

INFLAMMATION FIGHTER TIP: *You can boost the inflammation-fighting power of any meal by simply adding a side salad full of colorful vegetables. Choose phytochemical-rich dark leafy greens like spinach and kale, add vitamin C–rich tomatoes and vitamin D–rich mushrooms, and top with inflammation-reducing fresh herbs.*

SERVES 4 | PREP TIME: 5 MINUTES | COOK TIME: 10 MINUTES

Scallops are an excellent low-calorie source of magnesium and potassium, which are important for decreasing your risk for diabetes and maintaining healthy blood pressure levels. Packed with inflammation-reducing omega-3 fatty acids, vitamin B_{12}, antioxidants, and protein, they can be seared, broiled, and baked in minutes. In this recipe they team up with folate-rich snap peas for a delicious, low-calorie entrée.

1. In a large skillet over medium-high heat, add 1 teaspoon of the olive oil, and swirl the pan to coat the bottom. Add the snap peas, red bell pepper, ⅛ teaspoon salt, and ⅛ teaspoon pepper, and sauté for 2 minutes. Transfer the snap peas and bell pepper to a bowl.

2. Add the shallots to the skillet and sauté for 1 minute, and then transfer to the bowl with the snap peas and bell peppers.

3. Pat scallops dry with paper towels. Sprinkle evenly with the remaining ⅛ teaspoon salt and ⅛ teaspoon pepper. Add 1 teaspoon of the oil to pan and swirl to coat. Add half of scallops to the pan and cook for 2 minutes. Turn and cook for 1 minute more or until desired doneness. Place the cooked scallops on a plate. Repeat with remaining 1 teaspoon oil and remaining scallops.

4. Serve the scallops with the vegetable mixture and the lemon wedges alongside.

PER SERVING: CALORIES: 223; CARBS: 13G; GLYCEMIC LOAD: 8; FIBER: 3G; SODIUM: 421MG; PROTEIN: 31G; FAT: 5G; SATURATED FAT: 1G

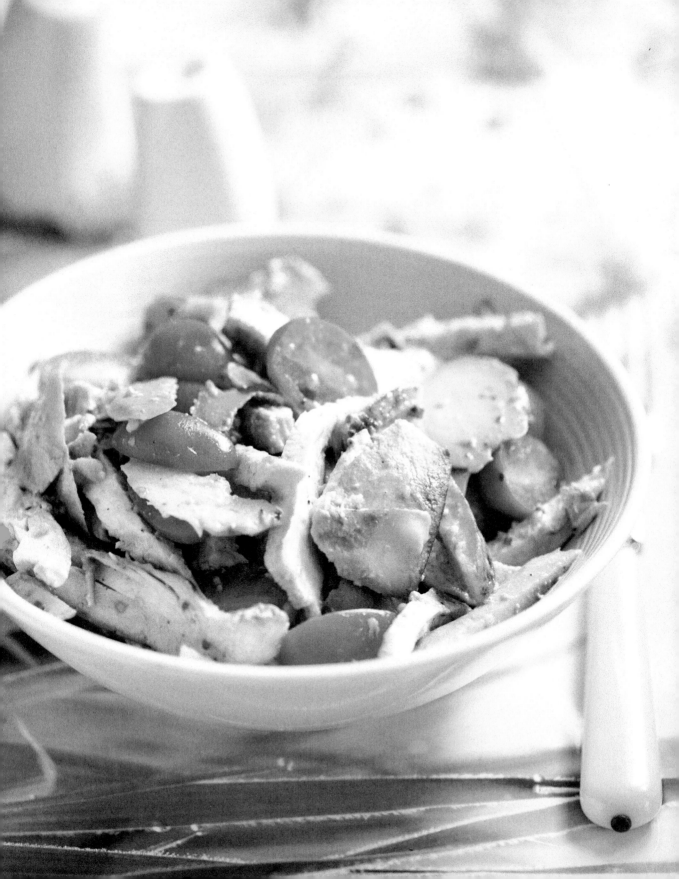

8

Poultry and Meat Entrées

Grilled Chicken and Avocado Salad

INFLAMMATION FIGHTER, GLUTEN FREE

FOR THE MARINADE

2 tablespoons plain nonfat
   Greek yogurt
2 tablespoons olive oil,
   divided
Juice of ½ lemon
4 garlic cloves, minced
1 teaspoon paprika
Salt
Freshly ground black pepper
1 pound boneless skinless
   chicken breast

FOR THE DRESSING

½ cup plain nonfat
   Greek yogurt
2 tablespoons
   red wine vinegar
1 tablespoon olive oil
1 garlic clove, minced

FOR THE SALAD

1 head butter lettuce,
   washed and torn
1 large avocado, pitted
   and cubed
½ red onion, thinly sliced
1 cup cherry
   tomatoes, halved
2 Persian cucumbers,
   thinly sliced

SERVES 4 | PREP TIME: 5 MINUTES, PLUS 20 MINUTES
TO MARINATE | COOK TIME: 10 MINUTES

*Packed with blood sugar–stabilizing protein, this delicious
grilled chicken and avocado salad delivers a healthy dose
of fiber, heart-healthy monounsaturated fats, free radical–
fighting vitamin C, and anti-inflammatory phytochemicals.
Plus, this simple recipe requires only a few staple ingredients
and can be easily customized by swapping in your favorite
vegetables.*

TO MAKE THE MARINADE

1. In a medium bowl, mix all the marinade ingredients
together.

2. Add the chicken, turning to coat on both sides. Cover
and refrigerate for 20 minutes.

3. When the chicken is done marinating, heat 1 tablespoon of the olive oil in a large skillet over high heat.
Place the marinated chicken in the skillet. Cook the
chicken for about 5 minutes per side, to an internal
temperature of 165°F. Remove the skillet from the heat.

TO MAKE THE DRESSING

Whisk together the dressing ingredients in a small bowl.

TO MAKE THE SALAD

1. Arrange the lettuce in 4 serving bowls and top with avocado, red onion, cherry tomatoes, and cucumber (if using).

2. Cut the chicken across the grain into thin slices. Divide among the 4 salads.

3. Pour the dressing over the 4 salads and season with salt and pepper.

LOWER CALORIE TIP: *This salad tastes terrific on its own without the salad dressing. To lower the calorie count, simply skip the dressing and season with salt, pepper, and red wine vinegar.*

PER SERVING: CALORIES: 357; CARBS: 15G; GLYCEMIC LOAD: 6; FIBER: 6G; SODIUM: 152MG; PROTEIN: 31G; FAT: 20G; SATURATED FAT: 4G

Chicken and Pepper Fajitas

FERTILITY BOOST, INFLAMMATION FIGHTER, DAIRY FREE, GLUTEN FREE

FOR THE MARINADE

1 tablespoon olive oil

2 tablespoons freshly
   squeezed lime juice

1½ teaspoons salt

1½ teaspoons dried oregano

1½ teaspoons ground cumin

1 teaspoon garlic powder

½ teaspoon chili powder

½ teaspoon paprika

½ teaspoon crushed red
   pepper flakes

FOR THE FAJITAS

1 pound free-range, organic
   boneless skinless
   chicken breasts, cut
   into ¼-inch-thick slices

1 tablespoon olive oil

2 red bell peppers, cut into
   thin strips

2 yellow or orange bell
   peppers, cut into
   thin strips

1 medium white onion, cut in
   half lengthwise, then sliced
   into thin half-moons

8 romaine lettuce leaves

2 tablespoons chopped fresh
   cilantro (optional)

SERVES 4 | PREP TIME: 15 MINUTES | COOK TIME: 11 MINUTES

Sure to be a family favorite, these healthy fajitas combine lean chicken strips, bell peppers, and onions, all served sizzling hot over romaine leaves. And the best part? You don't need to spend hours over the stove cooking, and no grilling is required. Chicken breast is best known for its protein content, but it is also an excellent source of B vitamins, including two that are especially important for fertility: folate and choline.

TO MAKE THE MARINADE

In a small bowl, whisk together the olive oil, lime juice, salt, oregano, cumin, garlic powder, chili powder, paprika, and red pepper flakes.

TO MAKE THE FAJITAS

1. Put the chicken slices into a large ziplock bag. Pour the marinade into the bag with the chicken. Seal the bag and set aside.

2. Heat the olive oil in a large skillet over medium-high heat. Add the red and yellow bell peppers and the onion, and sauté until the peppers are tender and the onion is turning translucent, about 4 minutes.

3. Transfer the peppers and onions to a large mixing bowl. Cover with foil to keep them warm.

4. In the same skillet over medium-high heat, sauté the chicken slices for 6 minutes, or until they are no longer pink. Return the bell pepper mixture to the pan and sauté to reheat, about 1 minute.

5. Serve the fajitas over the romaine leaves, and top with the cilantro (if using).

INFLAMMATION FIGHTER TIP: *You could boost the inflammation-fighting power of this recipe by adding freshly chopped tomatoes on top of your fajitas. Tomatoes are an excellent source of vitamin C, as well as the phytonutrient lycopene, which has been shown to reduce oxidative stress in the body. Choose tomatoes with rich colors to reap the most nutritional benefits.*

PER SERVING: CALORIES: 233; CARBS: 10G; GLYCEMIC LOAD: 3; FIBER: 3G; SODIUM: 661MG; PROTEIN: 27G; FAT: 9G; SATURATED FAT: 1G

Healthy and Easy Chicken Nuggets

LOWER CALORIE, DAIRY FREE, GLUTEN FREE

Olive oil cooking spray
1 pound, boneless skinless
   chicken breast, cut into
   bite-size chunks
2 teaspoons olive oil
½ teaspoon salt
½ teaspoon freshly ground
   black pepper
¼ cup almond flour
1 teaspoon garlic powder
1 teaspoon paprika
Olive oil cooking spray

SERVES 4 | PREP TIME: 10 MINUTES | COOK TIME: 15 MINUTES

It is tempting to go through the fast food drive-through when you need to put dinner on the table in a flash. Luckily, eating a whole food–based, minimally processed diet, requires less time than most people think. Grain-free and dairy-free, these easy baked chicken nuggets are fast, frugal, healthy, tasty, and kid-friendly. Plus, they get an extra kick of high-quality protein from their coating of vitamin E–rich almond flour. Serve them over a veggie salad for the adults and with crispy zucchini fries for the kids (see Cooking Tip).

1. Preheat the oven to 425°F.

2. Coat a baking sheet with olive oil cooking spray.

3. Put the chicken in a medium bowl. Add the olive oil and toss to coat the chicken. Season with the salt and pepper and toss once more.

4. In a second medium bowl, whisk together the almond flour, garlic powder, and paprika.

5. Drop a few chicken chunks at a time into the flour mixture to coat, then transfer them to the prepared baking sheet. Repeat with the remaining chicken chunks.

6. Lightly spray the top of the coated chicken chunks with olive oil cooking spray.

7. Bake for 10 minutes. Turn the chicken chunks over and cook for another 4 minutes, or until an instant-read meat thermometer inserted into a larger piece reads 165°F.

8. Remove the chicken nuggets from the oven and serve hot.

COOKING TIP: *While you are coating the chicken with the flour mixture, consider making a kid-pleasing side of vegetable fries. Simply slice zucchini, carrots, or another favorite vegetable into thin slices and coat them in a similar fashion as the chicken nuggets. Place the coated vegetables on a separate prepared baking sheet and bake until they are golden and tender, about 15 minutes.*

PER SERVING: CALORIES: 153; CARBS: 0G; GLYCEMIC LOAD: 0; FIBER: 0G; SODIUM: 364MG; PROTEIN: 26G; FAT: 4G; SATURATED FAT: 1G

Asian Chicken Lettuce Wraps

LOWER CALORIE, DAIRY FREE, GLUTEN FREE

FOR THE SAUCE

6 tablespoons low-sodium
   gluten-free soy sauce
   (or Bragg's liquid aminos)
2 garlic cloves, minced
1 tablespoon honey
2 tablespoons water
1 tablespoon peeled
   and finely chopped
   fresh ginger
1 tablespoon rice vinegar
1 tablespoon chili paste
Juice of 2 limes
1 teaspoon arrowroot powder

FOR THE CHICKEN WRAPS

1 tablespoon olive oil
1 pound ground
   chicken breast
8 green onions, chopped
1 (8-ounce) can water
   chestnuts, drained, rinsed,
   and chopped fine
1 red bell pepper,
   chopped fine
1 medium zucchini, trimmed
   and chopped fine
1 cup mushrooms, sliced
16 leaves butter lettuce,
   washed, for wrapping
1 carrot, peeled and grated,
   for topping (optional)
2 tablespoons finely chopped
   fresh cilantro, for topping
   (optional)
2 tablespoons coarsely
   chopped cashews, for
   topping (optional)

SERVES 4 | PREP TIME: 5 MINUTES | COOK TIME: 15 MINUTES

This simple and nutritious recipe is the perfect combination of savory, spicy, tangy, and sweet. Lean, protein-rich ground chicken is sautéed with vegetables, seasoned with Asian spices, and then served in a crispy lettuce leaf. Using lettuce leaves as wraps eliminates the need to use processed, high-carb tortillas; lowers the calories of the recipe; and adds fiber, vitamins A and C, and folate. Fun to eat, these wraps can be prepared in under 20 minutes.

TO MAKE THE SAUCE

In a small bowl, add the soy sauce, garlic, honey, water, ginger, rice vinegar, chili paste, lime juice, and arrowroot powder, whisk to combine. Set aside.

TO MAKE THE CHICKEN WRAPS

1. In a large skillet, heat the olive oil over medium-high heat. Add the chicken and brown until cooked through, about 8 minutes, sautéing with a wooden spoon and breaking up the pieces. Transfer the chicken to a paper towel–lined plate to drain the fat.

2. In the skillet, add the green onions, water chestnuts, red bell pepper, zucchini, and mushrooms, and sauté for 3 to 5 minutes until soft.

3. Return the chicken to the pan, add the sauce, and cook, stirring, for 2 minutes more.

4. With a slotted spoon, scoop the chicken mixture into the lettuce leaves. Top with the carrot, cilantro, or cashews (if using), and serve hot.

INFLAMMATION FIGHTER TIP: *Taking small but significant steps every day to build healthier eating habits is a long-term investment in your health and, when cooking for others, the health of your family. When you are making dinner, there isn't anything that says you can't double the amount of veggies a recipe calls for. Better yet, think varieties. If the recipe calls for red peppers, also add yellow. If it calls for spinach, then also add kale.*

PER SERVING: CALORIES: 351; CARBS: 34G; GLYCEMIC LOAD: 19; FIBER: 2G; SODIUM: 1590MG; PROTEIN: 26G; FAT: 13G; SATURATED FAT: 3G

Chicken Enchilada–Stuffed Spaghetti Squash

FERTILITY BOOST, INFLAMMATION FIGHTER, DAIRY FREE, GLUTEN FREE

2 small spaghetti squashes

2 tablespoons olive oil, divided

½ pound ground chicken breast

1 cup diced white onion

3 garlic cloves, minced

1 red bell pepper, finely chopped

1 cup cooked black beans, drained and rinsed

1 tablespoon cumin powder

1 tablespoon chili powder

1 tablespoon ground coriander

1 teaspoon salt

1 (8-ounce) can tomato sauce

¼ cup chopped fresh cilantro

1 chopped avocado, for topping (optional)

SERVES 4 | PREP TIME: 15 MINUTES | COOK TIME: 60 MINUTES

This recipe is packed full of healthy ingredients without compromising on flavor. The low carbohydrate spaghetti squash is rich in B vitamins, including folate, which supports the formation and development of new cells and may help prevent birth defects, making this squash an ideal food for pregnant women. This yellow vegetable is also high in the mineral potassium, which helps regulate blood pressure, and contains significant levels of omega-3 fats, which can reduce inflammation. Filled with protein-rich chicken, beans, and vegetables, this dish is hearty and satisfying without being overly heavy.

1. Preheat the oven to 425°F. Line a baking sheet with aluminum foil.

2. Cut the spaghetti squashes in half lengthwise and scrape out the seeds. Place the squash cut-side down in the prepared pan. Bake for 40 minutes or until the squash is easily pierced with the tip of a sharp knife. Remove the baking sheet from the oven and transfer the squash to a cooling rack.

3. Heat 1 tablespoon of the oil in a large skillet over medium-high heat. Add the chicken and brown until cooked through, about 8 minutes, stirring with a wooden spoon and breaking up the pieces. Transfer the cooked chicken to a paper towel–lined plate to drain.

4. Heat the remaining tablespoon of olive oil in the same skillet, add the onion, and sauté for 3 minutes. Add the garlic, reduce the heat to medium, and sauté for 3 minutes, until the garlic becomes fragrant and golden. Turn down the heat to medium low, add the bell pepper, and cook, stirring occasionally, for 5 minutes. Add the beans, chicken, cumin, chili powder, coriander, salt, and tomato sauce, and bring the mixture to a simmer. Turn off the heat and stir in the cilantro.

5. Using a fork, scrape and fluff the flesh of the squash, loosening it from the sides. Evenly divide the meat-vegetable mixture among the 4 halves, mounding it in the center.

6. Return the stuffed squashes to the oven and bake for 10 minutes more, until heated through.

7. Serve sprinkled with some cilantro and chopped avocado (if using).

INGREDIENT TIP: *The flesh of spaghetti squash possesses an uncanny resemblance to spaghetti strands when cooked, which is how it got its name. It can be added to a variety of dishes, such as soups or stews, or used as a pasta replacement and topped with pasta sauce. Low in carbohydrates and calories and rich in nutrients, this squash is a good choice to include in your diet.*

PER SERVING: CALORIES: 311; CARBS: 35G; GLYCEMIC LOAD: 12; FIBER: 6G; SODIUM: 660MG; PROTEIN: 16G; FAT: 13G; SATURATED FAT: 3G

Rosemary and Almond-Crusted Baked Chicken

INFLAMMATION FIGHTER, DAIRY FREE, GLUTEN FREE

1 pound boneless, skinless
   chicken breasts
Salt
Freshly ground black pepper
1 cup raw almonds
4 sprigs fresh rosemary,
   stemmed
1 tablespoon olive oil
1 medium shallot, minced
2 garlic cloves, minced
2 eggs

LOWER CALORIE TIP:
*To reduce the calories in this
recipe, you could replace
the eggs with unsweetened
almond milk. Submerge the
chicken in a bowl of milk
before coating it in the almond
mixture. You could also lightly
coat the chicken breasts with
olive oil cooking spray.*

SERVES 4 | PREP TIME: 10 MINUTES | COOK TIME: 40 MINUTES

*These baked chicken breasts are delicious and easy to
prepare with just a few staple ingredients. The almonds add
healthy fats and vitamin E, and the rosemary contributes
inflammation-fighting phytochemicals. To make this dish a
meal, consider serving it with a side of steamed green beans.*

1. Preheat the oven to 400°F with the oven rack in the
middle. Line a baking sheet with parchment paper.

2. Season the chicken breasts generously with salt and
pepper on both sides. Set aside.

3. In a food processor (or blender), chop the almonds
and rosemary until the mixture resembles coarse
crumbs. Transfer to a plate.

4. Heat the olive oil in a medium skillet over medium
heat. Add the shallot and garlic and sauté until soft, 2 to
3 minutes. Add the rosemary-almond mixture and cook,
stirring frequently, until golden brown, 5 to 10 minutes.
Transfer to a small, shallow bowl.

5. In another small, shallow bowl, beat the eggs,
dredge the chicken in the egg, then dredge it in the
rosemary-almond mixture. Press the crumbs to adhere to
the chicken.

6. Bake until golden brown and cooked through, and
the internal temperature is 165°F, about 25 minutes.
Serve warm.

PER SERVING: CALORIES: 403; CARBS: 8G; GLYCEMIC LOAD: 1; FIBER: 4G;
SODIUM: 143MG; PROTEIN: 37G; FAT: 26G; SATURATED FAT: 3G

Chicken and White Bean Chili

LOWER CALORIE, INFLAMMATION FIGHTER, DAIRY FREE

1 pound boneless, skinless chicken breast,

4 cups low-sodium chicken broth

2 cups chopped Vidalia onion

1 fresh medium jalapeño pepper, seeded and minced

2 garlic cloves, minced

1 (15-ounce) can cannellini beans, drained and rinsed

1 (4-ounce) can diced jalapeño chiles, with liquid

2 cups kale, stemmed and finely chopped

1 tablespoon ground cumin

1 teaspoon oregano

1 teaspoon salt

1 teaspoon freshly ground black pepper

⅓ cup chopped fresh cilantro

SERVES 8 | PREP TIME: 15 MINUTES | COOK TIME: 25 MINUTES

Who can say no to a bowl of warm, thick chili that's loaded with tender chicken and hearty cannellini beans? High in inflammation-fighting phytochemicals and vitamin C from the onions and peppers, and rich in B vitamins and blood sugar–balancing fiber from the beans, this high-protein chili has just enough kick and is ready in 30 minutes.

1. In a large heavy-bottomed soup pot or Dutch oven over medium-high heat, add the chicken and the chicken broth, bring the broth to a simmer, reduce the heat to medium, and cook until the chicken is tender, about 15 minutes.

2. Transfer the chicken to a plate and shred with two forks, then add back to the broth.

3. To the pot, add the onion, fresh jalapeño chile, garlic, beans, canned jalapeño chiles, kale, cumin, oregano, salt, and pepper. Stir well to combine. Turn down the heat to low, and simmer for about 10 minutes, until the vegetables are tender.

4. Serve hot, topped with the cilantro.

FERTILITY BOOST TIP: *For a one-pot chili meal that is higher in folate and choline, add 1 cup of cauliflower florets and consider doubling the quantity of beans used. Cannellini beans are a very good source of folate and are also high in vitamin C, an important antioxidant.*

PER SERVING: CALORIES: 165; CARBS: 19G; GLYCEMIC LOAD: 8; FIBER: 4G; SODIUM: 746MG; PROTEIN: 19G; FAT: 2G; SATURATED FAT: 0G

Turkey Meatballs over Greens

INFLAMMATION FIGHTER, DAIRY FREE, GLUTEN FREE

1 pound 93% to 97% lean
  ground turkey
¼ cup grated onion
1 cup grated zucchini
¼ cup flaxseed meal
1 egg, beaten
2 garlic cloves, minced
1 teaspoon salt
½ teaspoon freshly ground
  black pepper
2 tablespoons chopped fresh
  flat-leaf parsley
2 tablespoons olive oil,
  divided
2 cups Simple Tomato Sauce
  (page 193) or 1 (15-ounce)
  can tomato sauce
2 pounds kale, stemmed and
  roughly chopped

SERVES 4 | PREP TIME: 10 MINUTES | COOK TIME: 20 MINUTES

Consider this recipe your spaghetti and meatballs without the pasta. Piled on a bed of nutrient-rich kale instead of pasta, this gluten-free turkey meatball recipe replaces traditional bread crumbs with a combination of grated zucchini for moistness and flaxseed meal to hold the meat mixture together. Ready in just minutes, this is a super satisfying dinner that is high in protein, provides several servings of veggies, and won't weigh you down.

1. In a large bowl, combine the turkey, onion, zucchini, flaxseed meal, egg, garlic, salt, pepper, and parsley. With your clean hands, mix until thoroughly combined.

2. Roll the meat mixture into 1¼-inch meatballs and put on a plate. You should have 26 to 30 meatballs.

3. Heat 1 tablespoon of the olive oil in a large lidded skillet over medium-high heat. When the oil is hot, add the meatballs and brown for 3 to 4 minutes on each side. You may need to cook the meatballs in batches. Use tongs to gently rotate the meatballs so they brown evenly.

4. Reduce the heat to low, add all the meatballs, add the tomato sauce, and cover the pan. Simmer the meatballs and sauce for 10 minutes, or until the meatballs are cooked through.

5. Meanwhile, heat the remaining tablespoon of olive oil in another large skillet over medium-high heat. Add the kale and gently sauté until wilted and tender, about 5 minutes. Turn off the heat and cover to keep the kale warm until the meatballs are done.

6. Put the greens in a large shallow serving bowl, top with the meatballs and sauce, and serve hot.

LOWER CALORIE TIP: *You can lower the calories in this recipe by baking the turkey meatballs instead of pan sautéing them. Preheat the oven to 425°F. Coat a baking sheet with olive oil cooking spray. Put the meatballs in the prepared pan, and bake for 10 to 15 minutes to an internal temperature of 165°F.*

PER SERVING: CALORIES: 457; CARBS: 38G; GLYCEMIC LOAD: 15; FIBER: 8G; SODIUM: 819MG; PROTEIN: 32G; FAT: 22G; SATURATED FAT: 4G

Open-Face Turkey Veggie Burgers

DAIRY FREE, GLUTEN FREE

1 pound extra-lean
   ground turkey
1 cup grated zucchini
½ cup finely chopped
   mushrooms
2 garlic cloves, minced
2 tablespoons chopped
   green onions
2 shallots, chopped
Salt
Freshly ground black pepper
2 teaspoons olive oil
6 romaine heart
   lettuce leaves
1 medium tomato, cut
   into 6 slices

SERVES 6 | PREP TIME: 5 MINUTES | COOK TIME: 15 MINUTES

This healthy turkey burger recipe uses extra-lean ground turkey, grated zucchini and chopped mushrooms, and plenty of garlic, onions, and shallots to ensure that you won't sacrifice any taste. Made with clean ingredients, these burgers provide a hefty dose of high-quality protein, a serving of vegetables, and a host of vitamins, minerals, and phytochemicals.

1. In a large mixing bowl, combine the turkey, zucchini, mushrooms, garlic, green onions, shallots, and season with salt and pepper. Shape into 6 patties.

2. The patties can be cooked on an outdoor grill, in a skillet, or under the oven broiler. To use a large skillet, put it over medium heat and add the olive oil. Warm the oil till it begins to shimmer. Add the turkey patties and cook for about 6 minutes on each side, or until an instant-read thermometer reads an internal temperature of 165°F.

3. Serve the patties over the romaine leaves topped with a tomato slice.

INGREDIENT TIP: *Ground turkey may sound like a better choice than ground red meat, but it can be tricky reading the labels to determine which cut is actually lean, especially when many brands of ground turkey combine both white and dark meat. Extra lean is 99 percent fat-free and will be the lowest in fat and calories.*

PER SERVING: CALORIES: 137; CARBS: 2G; GLYCEMIC LOAD: 1; FIBER: 1G; SODIUM: 90MG; PROTEIN: 14G; FAT: 8G; SATURATED FAT: 2G

Herb-Roasted Turkey Breast

LOWER CALORIE, INFLAMMATION FIGHTER, DAIRY FREE, GLUTEN FREE

Olive oil cooking spray
1 pound boneless skinless
   turkey breast,
1 tablespoon olive oil
2 teaspoons freshly squeezed
   lemon juice
½ teaspoon freshly ground
   black pepper
¼ teaspoon salt
3 garlic cloves, minced into
   a paste
1 teaspoon chopped
   fresh thyme
1 teaspoon chopped
   fresh sage
1 teaspoon chopped
   fresh rosemary
1 teaspoon chopped fresh
   flat-leaf parsley
⅓ cup water

INGREDIENT TIP: *Using fresh or dried herbs in a recipe really depends on your preference, and often the decision is based purely on what the cook has available. Dried herbs are more potent than fresh. A good rule-of-thumb conversion is 1 tablespoon fresh equals 1 teaspoon dried.*

SERVES 4 | PREP TIME: 5 MINUTES | COOK TIME: 40 MINUTES

Skinless white-meat turkey is rich in protein, low in fat, and has a very low GI. High in B vitamins, iron, zinc, and potassium, turkey is a great source of the neurotransmitter serotonin, which plays a role in the regulation of mood and appetite. Serve this nutritious dish with a side of steamed vegetables and a green salad.

1. Preheat the oven to 350°F. Coat a 9-by-13-inch baking dish with olive oil cooking spray.

2. Lay the turkey breast in the prepared pan and lightly spray both sides with olive oil.

3. In a small bowl, combine the olive oil, lemon juice, pepper, salt, garlic, thyme, sage, rosemary, and parsley and stir well to mix thoroughly. Rub the mixture into both sides of the turkey breast. Coat the top with olive oil cooking spray.

4. Carefully pour the water in the bottom of the baking dish to keep the turkey moist. Cover with foil and bake for 30 to 40 minutes or until an instant-read meat thermometer registers 165°F degrees when inserted into the thickest part of a turkey breast.

5. Remove the turkey from the oven and place the baking dish on a wire rack to rest for 10 minutes, keeping it covered with foil.

6. Slice the turkey and serve hot.

PER SERVING: CALORIES: 158; CARBS: 1G; GLYCEMIC LOAD: 0; FIBER: 0G; SODIUM: 201MG; PROTEIN: 28G; FAT: 4G; SATURATED FAT: 1G

Quick Pan-Seared Turkey Cutlets

LOW CALORIE, DAIRY FREE, GLUTEN FREE

2 tablespoons
 olive oil, divided
2 tablespoons freshly
 squeezed lemon juice
1 teaspoon tarragon
1 teaspoon garlic powder
1 pound turkey cutlets
Salt
Freshly ground black pepper

SERVES 4 | PREP TIME: 5 MINUTES | COOK TIME: 10 MINUTES

One advantage of turkey cutlets is that they cook quickly. They are also low in fat and high in protein, B vitamins, and iron. In this recipe, the cutlets are seasoned with lemon and tarragon, an herb rich in vitamins A and C along with inflammation-fighting phytochemicals. Crispy on the outside and juicy on the inside, these cutlets are delicious over a salad or with a side of steamed vegetables.

1. In a shallow dish, whisk 1 tablespoon of the olive oil, lemon juice, tarragon, and garlic powder.

2. Season the turkey cutlets with salt and pepper, and dredge in the oil-herb mix.

3. Heat the remaining tablespoon of olive oil in a large skillet over medium-high heat. Working in batches, cook cutlets until browned and opaque throughout, 2 to 3 minutes per side. The outside should be nicely browned and the inside fully cooked and opaque, to a meat thermometer reading of 165°F.

4. Let the turkey rest a few minutes before serving.

INGREDIENT TIP: *Tarragon has a subtle but pronounced taste, which goes well with artichokes, asparagus, Brussels sprouts, cauliflower, and carrots. Choose your favorite of these vegetables to steam as a side to this dish, and season them with a tarragon vinaigrette (1 to 2 tablespoons of fresh tarragon, white wine vinegar, and olive oil).*

PER SERVING: CALORIES: 184; CARBS: 0G; GLYCEMIC LOAD: 0; FIBER: 0G; SODIUM: 79MG; PROTEIN: 28G; FAT: 7G; SATURATED FAT: 1G

Slow Cooker Turkey Breast with Rosemary and Garlic

LOWER CALORIE, INFLAMMATION FIGHTER, DAIRY FREE, GLUTEN FREE

Olive oil cooking spray
1 cup chopped white onion
1 cup sliced carrots
1 cup halved Brussels sprouts
1 tablespoon minced garlic
1 teaspoon chopped
    fresh rosemary
1 teaspoon chopped
    fresh sage
1 teaspoon chopped fresh
    flat-leaf parsley
1 teaspoon paprika
1 tablespoon olive oil
1 tablespoon freshly
    squeezed lemon juice
Salt
Freshly ground black pepper
2 pounds boneless skinless
    turkey breast

INFLAMMATION FIGHTER TIP: *You can add to the inflammation-fighting power of this meal by serving it with sautéed mixed greens, such as kale, spinach, and Swiss chard. Try to get into the habit of having at least one serving of dark leafy greens each day to boost your intake of vitamins A and C and important phytochemicals.*

SERVES 4 | PREP TIME: 10 MINUTES| COOK TIME: 4 TO 6 HOURS ON HIGH, OR 7 TO 10 HOURS ON LOW

Not only are Brussels sprouts a great source of antioxidants, but they contain vitamin K, glucosinolates, and alpha-linolenic acid, three key nutrients that have been shown to help regulate and prevent unwanted inflammation in the body. Paired with turkey breast and a variety of vegetables and herbs, they create a healthy dinner that's perfect for even the busiest weeknight.

1. Coat the inside of a slow cooker insert with olive oil cooking spray.

2. In the bottom of the insert, arrange the onion, carrots, Brussels sprouts, and garlic.

3. In a small bowl, mix the garlic, rosemary, sage, parsley, paprika, olive oil, lemon juice, salt, and pepper. Brush the seasoning mixture over the turkey breast.

4. Add the turkey to the slow cooker, placing it on top of the vegetables.

5. Cook on high for 4 to 6 hours or on low for 7 to 10 hours, until the turkey is cooked through. Check the internal temperature with an instant-read meat thermometer to make sure it is 165°F before serving.

6. Remove the turkey from the slow cooker and slice it thinly across the grain. Divide the sliced turkey and slow-cooked vegetables among 4 plates; serve hot.

PER SERVING: CALORIES: 320; CARBS: 9G; GLYCEMIC LOAD: 3; FIBER: 2G; SODIUM: 164MG; PROTEIN: 57G; FAT: 5G; SATURATED FAT: 1G

Stir-Fried Pork and Vegetables

LOWER CALORIE, INFLAMMATION FIGHTER, DAIRY FREE, GLUTEN FREE

FOR THE PORK

4 (4-ounce) boneless pork
   loin chops, sliced into
   2-inch-long thin strips
2 teaspoons arrowroot powder
1½ tablespoons gluten-free
   low-sodium soy sauce, or
   Bragg's liquid aminos

FOR THE SAUCE

1½ tablespoons gluten-free
   low-sodium soy sauce, or
   Bragg's liquid aminos
Juice of ½ lime
½ teaspoon honey
1 teaspoon toasted sesame oil
2 teaspoons rice vinegar
2 teaspoons Sriracha sauce

FOR THE STIR-FRY

2 teaspoons olive oil
2 teaspoons peeled and grated
   fresh ginger
4 garlic cloves, crushed
1 cup snow peas
½ cup shredded
   purple cabbage
1 cup sliced shiitake
   mushrooms
1 medium red bell
   pepper, sliced
1 medium yellow summer
   squash, sliced
¼ cup sliced green onions,
   for garnish

SERVES 4 | PREP TIME: 10 MINUTES | COOK TIME: 15 MINUTES

Stir-fry dishes are a great choice for busy weeknight dinners, because they are quick to prepare and you can use any combination of protein and vegetables. This recipe uses vitamin B–rich pork and a mix of antioxidant-rich vegetables given a slightly spicy kick from the addition of Sriracha sauce. This recipe is satisfying enough on its own, so no rice is used keeping the carb content high in fiber and quality from veggies only.

TO MAKE THE PORK

Put the pork chops in a medium-size baking dish. In a small bowl, combine the arrowroot and soy sauce. Set aside.

TO MAKE THE SAUCE

In a small bowl, combine the soy sauce, lime juice, honey, sesame oil, vinegar, and Sriracha sauce, whisk to mix well, and set aside.

TO MAKE THE STIR-FRY

1. Heat a large skillet over high heat. Add 1 teaspoon of the oil and the pork and sauté 6 to 7 minutes until browned. Transfer to a plate and set aside.

2. To the skillet, add the remaining 1 teaspoon olive oil, ginger, garlic, snow peas, cabbage, mushrooms, bell pepper, and squash. Reduce the heat to low, and pour the sauce over the vegetables. Sauté for 2 minutes.

3. Return the pork to the pan and sauté to reheat, 2 to 3 minutes.

4. Top with the green onions, and serve hot

FERTILITY BOOST TIP: *To boost the folate in this recipe, use 1 cup of trimmed and chopped asparagus spears in addition to or in place of the yellow summer squash. Serving this dish over riced cauliflower would add choline, a nutrient important for reducing the risk of harmful gene effects that could result in birth defects.*

PER SERVING: CALORIES: 200; CARBS: 11G; GLYCEMIC LOAD: 6; FIBER: 2G; SODIUM: 879MG; PROTEIN: 27G; FAT: 5G; SATURATED FAT: 2G

Walnut-Crusted Pork Tenderloin

LOWER CALORIE, DAIRY FREE, GLUTEN FREE

1 pound pork tenderloin
1 tablespoon mustard powder
1 tablespoon ground sage
1 tablespoon ground
　rosemary
1 tablespoon paprika
1 tablespoon onion powder
1 tablespoon garlic powder
1 teaspoon salt
1½ teaspoons freshly ground
　black pepper
½ cup walnuts

INFLAMMATION FIGHTER TIP: *Pair your nut-crusted pork tenderloin with a mix of cruciferous vegetables for maximum nutrition and inflammation-fighting power. Brussels sprouts, broccoli, cauliflower, cabbage, collards, and kale are just a few types of these vegetables, which contain important phytochemicals, vitamins, minerals, and fiber. Select a mix and steam them for a healthy side dish.*

SERVES 4 | PREP TIME: 10 MINUTES | COOK TIME: 30 MINUTES

This recipe uses one of the healthiest pork options, the tenderloin. Lean cuts of pork are high in protein, are low in fat, and have more B vitamins than many other types of meat. These vitamins play a role in a variety of bodily functions, including metabolism and energy production. Pork is also high in high in the antioxidant minerals and selenium. Serve this simple yet nutritious pork tenderloin with a salad or mixed greens and steamed vegetables.

1. Preheat the oven to 375°F.

2. Pat the tenderloin dry with a paper towel.

3. In a small bowl, mix the mustard powder, sage, rosemary, paprika, onion powder, garlic powder, salt, and pepper. Rub the pork tenderloin evenly with the spice mixture.

4. In a food processor (or blender), pulse the walnuts until finely chopped. Coat the pork tenderloin evenly with the chopped walnuts.

5. Place the tenderloin in a baking pan and cook for 30 minutes, or until the internal temperature on a meat thermometer reads 145°F.

6. Let the pork rest for 10 minutes. Cut into slices crosswise, and serve hot.

PER SERVING: CALORIES: 230; CARBS: 2G; GLYCEMIC LOAD: 0; FIBER: 1G; SODIUM: 640MG; PROTEIN: 25G; FAT: 13G; SATURATED FAT: 2G

Italian Baked Pork Chops with Fennel and Green Beans

INFLAMMATION FIGHTER, DAIRY FREE, GLUTEN FREE

4 tablespoons olive oil, divided

3 tablespoons freshly squeezed lemon juice

2 tablespoons chopped fresh basil

1 teaspoon ground oregano

4 garlic cloves, chopped

Salt

Freshly ground black pepper

4 bone-in pork loin chops, ½ inch thick

1 fennel bulb, cut into 8 pieces (see Cooking Tip)

3 cups trimmed greens beans

3 jarred roasted red bell peppers, drained and coarsely chopped

COOKING TIP: *The three different parts of fennel—the bulb, stalks, and leaves—can all be used in cooking. Cut the stalks away from the bulb at the place where they meet. If you are not going to be using the intact bulb in a recipe, then first cut it in half, remove the base, and then rinse it with water before proceeding to cut it further. The stalks of the fennel can be used for soups, stocks, and stews, while the leaves can be used as an herb seasoning.*

SERVES 4 | PREP TIME: 5 MINUTES | COOK TIME: 30 MINUTES

This inflammation-fighting baked pork chop gets a phytonutrient boost from the fennel bulb. High in fiber, vitamin C, folate, and potassium, this vegetable has a unique combination of phytonutrients that give it strong antioxidant activity that may reduce inflammation in the body. With several servings of vegetables, this high protein dish is certain to please.

1. Preheat the oven to 475°F.

2. In a large bowl, mix 2 tablespoons of the olive oil, the lemon juice, basil, oregano, and garlic, and season with salt and black pepper. Add the pork chops and turn to coat.

3. On a large baking sheet, toss the fennel bulb, green beans, and red bell peppers with the remaining 2 tablespoons olive oil, and season with salt and black pepper. Spread in an even layer.

4. Nestle the pork chops among the vegetables. Roast for 30 minutes, turning the pork chops once halfway through the cooking time, until the vegetables are tender and the pork chops are cooked through, or to an internal temperature of 145°F.

5. Serve hot.

PER SERVING: CALORIES: 330; CARBS: 17G; GLYCEMIC LOAD: 6; FIBER: 7G; SODIUM: 98MG; PROTEIN: 26G; FAT: 18G; SATURATED FAT: 3G

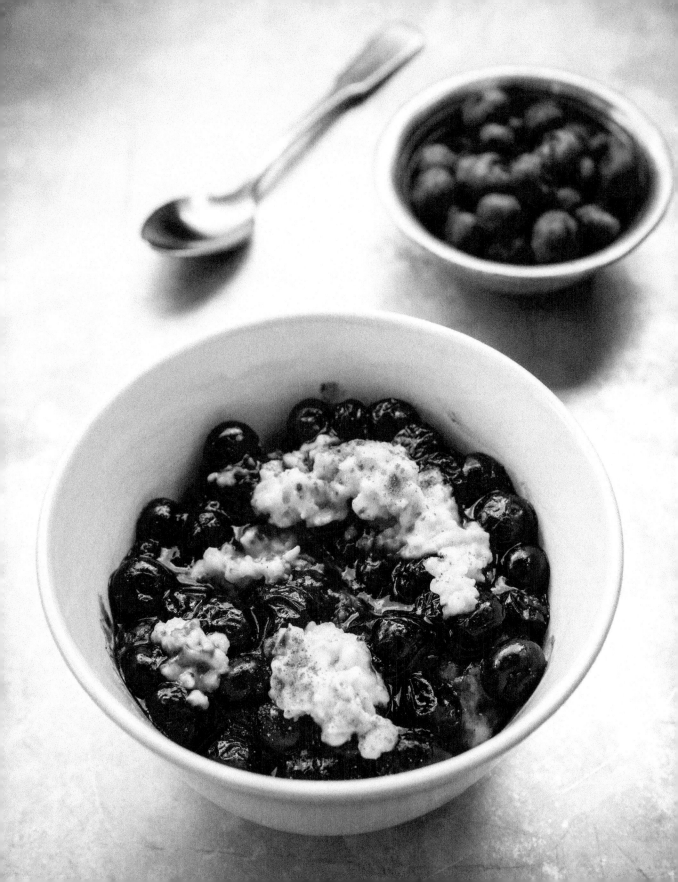

9

Drinks and Desserts

Iced Ginger Chai

LOWER CALORIE, INFLAMMATION FIGHTER, DAIRY FREE, GLUTEN FREE

12 cardamom pods,
   gently crushed
8 whole black peppercorns
8 whole cloves
4-inch piece fresh ginger,
   peeled and sliced
4 cups water
4 cinnamon sticks
1 teaspoon powdered stevia
2 star anise
1 vanilla bean, sliced down
   the middle
⅛ teaspoon ground nutmeg
4 black tea bags

INFLAMMATION
FIGHTER TIP: *Teas are an
extremely rich source of natural
antioxidants and phytochemicals. Because each type of
tea has its own unique set of
nutrients, there is really no one
best choice. Consider trying a
variety of different types in this
recipe, including black, white,
red (rooibos), and even herbal
types such as chamomile
and ginger.*

SERVES 8 (4 CUPS CONCENTRATE) | PREP TIME: 5 MINUTES
COOK TIME: 20 MINUTES

*If you are in love with the delicious chai drinks sold at coffee
shops, but can't tolerate the sugar content or the prices,
consider making homemade chai concentrate. All you need
is a handful of spices and seasonings and about 20 minutes
of cooking time to prepare a batch that you can use throughout the week. You can also tweak the recipe according to
your preferences and make it more peppery or sweeter by
varying the quantities of the ingredients. Experiment until
you find the taste that is right for you. If you want to make
a caffeine-free version of this concentrate, use 4 bags of
rooibos tea instead of the black tea.*

1. In a large saucepan over medium-high heat, stir
together the cardamom, peppercorns, cloves, ginger,
water, cinnamon sticks, stevia, star anise, vanilla bean,
and nutmeg. Bring the mixture to a boil, reduce the heat
to low, cover, and simmer for 15 minutes. Add the tea
bags, cover, remove the pan from the heat, and let the
mixture steep for 5 minutes.

2. Set a fine-mesh strainer over a large bowl. Pour the
tea mixture through the strainer. Discard the solids and
let the concentrated liquid cool to room temperature.
Pour the concentrate into glass jars and refrigerate
until chilled.

3. To serve, mix equal parts concentrate and cold water
or milk to make chai tea. Refrigerate in an airtight container for up to 1 week.

PER SERVING: CALORIES: 3; CARBS: 1G; GLYCEMIC LOAD: 0; FIBER: 0G;
SODIUM: 0MG; PROTEIN: 0G; FAT: 0G; SATURATED FAT: 0G

Homemade Quinoa Milk

LOWER CALORIE, DAIRY FREE, GLUTEN FREE

1 cup cooked quinoa

3 cups filtered water, divided

3 Medjool dates, pitted, soaked, and chopped

1 teaspoon vanilla extract

Pinch salt

¼ teaspoon ground cinnamon (optional)

INFLAMMATION FIGHTER TIP: *For a tasty boost, add 2 tablespoons walnuts, ½ teaspoon peeled and grated fresh ginger, and 1 additional pitted date. The resulting walnut-ginger quinoa milk will have added omega-3 fats and gingerols for reducing inflammation.*

SERVES 4 | PREP TIME: 15 MINUTES

This protein-rich beverage can be used in smoothies, poured over granola, and so much more. It is incredibly easy to make yourself. You will need a piece of cheesecloth, which is sold in pretty much every large grocery store. Once you make the basic recipe, you can bump up the flavor with additional dates or coconut sugar, a dash of cinnamon, or even a few cacao nibs or tablespoons of cocoa powder. Quinoa is a complete protein, rich in inflammation-reducing phytochemicals, making this a perfect beverage to include in your diet.

1. In a blender, combine the quinoa and 1 cup of the water; blend on high for 1 to 3 minutes until smooth.

2. Put a large sieve over a large bowl and line it with three layers of cheesecloth. Pour the quinoa milk into the cheesecloth over the bowl. The milk will strain slowly on its own, but you can gently squeeze and massage the bottom of the cheesecloth to speed up the process.

3. Put the strained quinoa milk back into the blender and add more of the water 1 cup at a time, blending the mixture after each addition until it reaches your desired consistency. Add the dates, vanilla, salt, and cinnamon (if using) and blend until smooth.

4. Store the milk in an airtight jar in the refrigerator for up to 3 days.

PER SERVING: CALORIES: 32; CARBS: 4G; GLYCEMIC LOAD: 2; FIBER: 0G; SODIUM: 25MG; PROTEIN: 0G; FAT: 0G; SATURATED FAT: 0G

Cucumber, Ginger, and Lime Mocktail

LOWER CALORIE, INFLAMMATION FIGHTER, DAIRY FREE, GLUTEN FREE

6 medium cucumbers

2 cups water

1-inch piece fresh ginger, peeled and sliced

½ teaspoon powdered stevia

6 tablespoons freshly squeezed lime juice

SERVES 6 | PREP TIME: 10 MINUTES, PLUS 2 HOURS TO CHILL

This deliciously refreshing, nonalcoholic beverage is akin to drinking liquid superfood. Ginger is full of antioxidants and anti-inflammatories and is known to reduce joint pain, promote digestion, and support a healthy immune system. Lime juice is packed with the antioxidant vitamin C and bioflavonoids. And the cool, refreshing taste of cucumber ties it all together, making this the perfect beverage for hot summer days.

1. Set a large strainer over a large bowl. Line it with several layers of cheesecloth or paper towels.

2. Trim the ends off the cucumbers. Cut 6 slices about ¼ inch thick to use for garnish; set aside on a plate. Peel the remaining cucumbers, halve them lengthwise, and scoop out the seeds. Cut into large pieces and transfer to a food processor (or blender); process until the cucumbers are reduced to pulp, about 2 minutes.

3. Pour the pulp into the prepared strainer and use a silicone spatula to press all the juice from the mixture.

4. In a medium saucepan over medium heat, combine the water, ginger, and stevia. Bring to a simmer and cook, stirring constantly, for about 5 minutes. Remove the pan from the heat; remove and discard the ginger slices. Stir in the lime juice.

5. Remove the strainer from the bowl and discard the cucumber pulp. Stir in the stevia-ginger mixture and set the mixture aside to cool to room temperature. Pour the drink into a large jar or pitcher and refrigerate until completely cooled, at least 2 hours.

6. Serve over ice cubes, garnishing each glass with a slice of cucumber.

INGREDIENT TIP: *Whenever possible, choose fresh ginger over dried and ground ginger. Not only does fresh ginger taste better, but it also contains higher levels of gingerol as well as ginger's active anti-inflammatory compound. Fresh ginger is sold in the produce section of most grocery stores. When purchasing, make sure it is firm, smooth, and free of mold.*

PER SERVING: CALORIES: 49; CARBS: 12G; GLYCEMIC LOAD: 3; FIBER: 2G; SODIUM: 6MG; PROTEIN: 2G; FAT: 0G; SATURATED FAT: 0G

Coconut Mango Smoothie

LOWER CALORIE, INFLAMMATION FIGHTER, DAIRY FREE, GLUTEN FREE

1 tablespoon chia seeds

½ cup water

1 cup unsweetened
almond milk

¼ cup canned light
coconut milk

¾ cup nonfat plain
Greek yogurt

1 tablespoon coconut flour

1 cup frozen mango

1 to 2 Medjool dates, pitted,
soaked, and chopped

½ teaspoon coconut extract
(optional)

1 cup ice

SERVES 2 | PREP TIME: 10 MINUTES

Smoothies done right make a healthy snack, breakfast, or even light lunch. The key is to include a mix of protein, fiber-rich carbs, and healthy fats to keep you feeling full and your blood sugar steady. This tropical smoothie is sweetened naturally with dates and contains high-quality protein from the Greek yogurt, plus antioxidants and vitamin C from the mango. Add a sprig of mint for the perfect garnish.

1. Place the chia seeds in a small bowl, cover them with the water, and refrigerate for 5 minutes. The chia seeds will soak up the water and form a gel.

2. Add the chia gel to a blender. Add the almond milk, coconut milk, yogurt, coconut flour, mango, dates, and coconut extract (if using). Add more or less ice to reach your desired consistency; process until smooth.

3. Immediately, pour into two tall glasses and serve.

INGREDIENT TIP: *Chia seeds add fiber, healthy fats, and protein to your smoothies, plus they make a great thickener. To make the gel, add 4 tablespoons chia seeds to 2 cups water. Let stand for 15 to 30 minutes at room temperature or refrigerate for 5 to 10 minutes, stirring occasionally to prevent clumping. The gel can be used as a thickener for smoothies, soups, and fresh jams.*

PER SERVING: CALORIES: 362; CARBS: 47G; GLYCEMIC LOAD: 19; FIBER: 6G; SODIUM: 145MG; PROTEIN: 9G; FAT: 18G; SATURATED FAT: 12G

Raspberry Almond Smoothie

INFLAMMATION FIGHTER, DAIRY FREE, GLUTEN FREE

1 cup unsweetened
    almond milk
¾ cup vanilla soy yogurt
    (or Greek yogurt)
1 frozen banana, sliced
1 cup frozen raspberries
1 tablespoon natural
    almond butter
2 teaspoons wheat germ
½ teaspoon vanilla extract
1 cup ice, or as desired

SERVES 2 | PREP TIME: 5 MINUTES

This creamy, delicious smoothie is a perfect post-workout snack or healthy dessert. Raspberries are one of the most nutritious fruits you can eat. They are very low in calories, and one cup offers a whopping 8 grams of dietary fiber, almost half of a day's recommended amount of vitamin C, and good amounts of phenolic phytochemicals that may play a role in reducing inflammation. With healthy fats from almond butter and wheat germ, this smoothie provides a balance of energizing and healing nutrients. If preferred, you can substitute Greek yogurt for the soy yogurt.

1. In a blender, combine the almond milk, yogurt, banana, raspberries, almond butter, wheat germ, and vanilla. Add more or less ice to reach your desired consistency; process until smooth.

2. Immediately, pour into two tall glasses and serve.

INGREDIENT TIP: *One key to making smoothies that won't spike your blood sugar is to always include a source of protein. While there are many dairy-free yogurt options, not all of them contain this important nutrient, so be certain to read the nutrition facts panel before making your decision. Avoid newer brands of yogurt that contain pea protein.*

PER SERVING: CALORIES: 331; CARBS: 59G; GLYCEMIC LOAD: 21; FIBER: 8G; SODIUM: 138MG; PROTEIN: 9G; FAT: 8G; SATURATED FAT: 2G

Peaches and Greens Smoothie

FERTILITY BOOST, INFLAMMATION FIGHTER, DAIRY FREE, GLUTEN FREE

1½ cups unsweetened
  almond milk
⅓ cup frozen edamame
½ cup thawed frozen spinach
1 cup frozen peaches
1 tablespoon hemp seeds
2 teaspoons tahini
  (sesame paste)
1 to 2 Medjool dates, pitted,
  soaked, and chopped
  (see Ingredient Tip)
1 cup ice, or as desired

SERVES 2 | PREP TIME: 5 MINUTES

This creamy and delicious, inflammation-fighting smoothie is made using vitamin C–rich peaches, protein-rich edamame, and the nutritional powerhouse spinach. Spinach is an excellent source of vitamin A, fertility-boosting folate, phytochemicals, B vitamins, and numerous minerals. The use of frozen fruits and vegetables creates a sweet, thick, and nutritious drink that can serve double duty as a dessert or healthy snack. If preferred, you can substitute the dates with powdered or liquid stevia, a lower-calorie option.

1. In a blender, combine the almond milk, edamame, spinach, peaches, hemp seeds, tahini, and dates. Add more or less ice to reach your desired consistency; process until smooth.

2. Immediately, pour into two tall glasses and serve.

INGREDIENT TIP: *Medjool dates allow you to add fiber, vitamins and minerals to your smoothie, sweeten it up, and avoid the use of processed or refined sugars all at the same time. Soak your dates first to allow for easier blending, and be certain that the pits have been removed.*

PER SERVING: CALORIES: 236; CARBS: 36G; GLYCEMIC LOAD: 14; FIBER: 5G; SODIUM: 118MG; PROTEIN: 8G; FAT: 9G; SATURATED FAT: 1G

Five-Minute Vegan Hot Cocoa

LOWER CALORIE, INFLAMMATION FIGHTER, DAIRY FREE, GLUTEN FREE

4 cups unsweetened almond milk
4 tablespoons unsweetened cocoa powder
½ teaspoon powdered stevia
¼ teaspoon ground cinnamon
½ teaspoon vanilla extract

SERVES 4 | PREP TIME: 1 MINUTE | COOK TIME: 4 MINUTES

This vegan hot chocolate is made with simple, healthy ingredients that you probably already have on hand. Cocoa contains flavonoids that aid in lowering blood pressure, as well as essential minerals like calcium and potassium. Sweetened with a natural plant-based sweetener, stevia, this drink will satisfy that chocolate craving without messing with your blood sugar levels.

1. Pour the almond milk into a large saucepan over medium heat and cook until it is just heated through, whisking often.

2. Add the cocoa powder, stevia, and cinnamon, and whisk vigorously to combine.

3. Continue cooking until the mixture is completely combined and the cocoa reaches the temperature you prefer.

4. Remove the pan from the heat. Taste and adjust the sweetness, if necessary. Stir in the vanilla.

5. Pour the cocoa into 4 mugs and serve immediately.

INGREDIENT TIP: *Cacao or cocoa, which is better? Both of them are unique when it comes to taste, nutrition, and cost. Cacao is a term used for the tree, pod, seeds, and cacao nibs; it is considered a raw food and is the purest form of chocolate you can consume. Cocoa is the processed form of cacao that you eat when you consume hot cocoa or a chocolate bar. Both are rich in antioxidants and make a good choice. You may consider giving both a try to see which you prefer.*

PER SERVING: CALORIES: 132; CARBS: 18G; GLYCEMIC LOAD: 4; FIBER: 3G; SODIUM: 280MG; PROTEIN: 3G; FAT: 5G; SATURATED FAT: 0G

Banana "Ice Cream"

LOWER CALORIE, DAIRY FREE, GLUTEN FREE

6 to 8 ripe bananas
(use 1 to 2 per person)
½ cup unsweetened
almond milk
1 teaspoon vanilla extract

OPTIONAL ADDITIONS:
ground cinnamon, cocoa
powder, minced
fresh ginger
Optional toppings: fresh
berries, sliced nuts,
chia seeds

SERVES 4 | PREP TIME: 5 MINUTES, PLUS AT LEAST 2 HOURS
TO FREEZE | PROCESSING TIME: 5 MINUTES

This simple recipe turns frozen bananas and almond milk into delicious soft-serve "ice cream" in minutes, with zero dairy or refined sugar. You can use a food processor or blender, though a food processor produces a creamier result. High in blood pressure–regulating potassium, this dessert is a worthy ice-cream contender.

1. Peel the bananas and slice them into coins. Put the bananas in an airtight container and freeze them for at least 2 hours, ideally overnight.

2. In a food processor (or blender), combine the frozen banana slices, almond milk, and vanilla.

3. Blend until smooth and creamy, taking two or three breaks to stir the mixture before blending again.

4. Immediately pour the "ice cream" into bowls and serve.

INGREDIENT TIP: *There are numerous ways to step up this treat. For an even creamier texture, use soy milk, canned light coconut milk, or 1 to 2 tablespoons of your favorite nut butter. Note that adding nut butter or other types of milk will raise the calorie count.*

PER SERVING: CALORIES: 190; CARBS: 47G; GLYCEMIC LOAD: 17; FIBER: 5G; SODIUM: 20MG; PROTEIN: 2G; FAT: 1G; SATURATED FAT: 0G

Baked Apples

LOWER CALORIE, INFLAMMATION FIGHTER, DAIRY FREE, GLUTEN FREE

2 large apples

1 teaspoon coconut oil

2 teaspoons powdered stevia

2 tablespoons almond meal or almond flour

4 tablespoons old-fashioned rolled oats

2 tablespoons unsweetened almond milk

¼ teaspoon ground cinnamon

Pinch ground nutmeg

SERVES 4 | PREP TIME: 5 MINUTES | COOK TIME: 30 MINUTES

Healthy desserts don't have to be complicated. In fact, when it comes to eating a diet of whole, unprocessed foods, simpler is always better. Here, phytonutrient- and fiber-rich apples are topped with oats and seasoned with cinnamon to create individual apple crisps without all of the fuss. A simple, low-fat, healthy dessert for a cool autumn evening.

1. Preheat the oven to 350°F.

2. Line a small baking pan with parchment paper.

3. Cut the apples in half, and remove and discard the core and seeds with a small paring knife or spoon.

4. In a small bowl, combine coconut oil, stevia, almond meal, oats, almond milk, and cinnamon. Spoon on top of the apple halves and sprinkle with the nutmeg.

5. Put the apples on the prepared pan and bake for 30 minutes.

6. Serve warm.

INFLAMMATION FIGHTER TIP: *For additional vitamin C, fiber, and phytochemicals, add 1 to 2 fresh cranberries on top of each apple before baking. Cranberries are very low in calories and offer powerful anti-inflammatory benefits due to their impressive array of proanthocyanidins, a type of phytonutrient.*

PER SERVING: CALORIES: 119; CARBS: 22G; GLYCEMIC LOAD: 7; FIBER: 4G; SODIUM: 10MG; PROTEIN: 2G; FAT: 3G; SATURATED FAT: 1G

Blueberry Porridge

INFLAMMATION FIGHTER, DAIRY FREE, GLUTEN FREE

1 cup uncooked millet
1 tablespoon chia seeds
½ cup slivered almonds,
  divided
1½ cups water
1½ cups unsweetened
  almond milk, plus more for
  serving (optional)
1 teaspoon vanilla extract
Pinch salt
1 cup frozen blueberries
1 to 2 teaspoons
  granulated stevia

INFLAMMATION FIGHTER TIP: *You can boost the inflammation-fighting power of this recipe by doubling the fruit. Add a cup of antioxidant-rich cherries or raspberries. Both of these berries are low-glycemic-index fruits rich in phytochemicals shown to reduce inflammation and the risk for chronic disease.*

SERVES 6 | PREP TIME: 5 MINUTES | COOK TIME: 20 MINUTES

Sometimes you need to think outside of the box. Hot cooked cereals don't just have to be served for breakfast, they also make nutrient-rich and satisfying desserts. This antioxidant-, protein-, and fiber-rich porridge uses the gluten-free seed, millet, along with the powerhouse fruit, blueberries. Sweetened with natural stevia and thickened with chia seeds, which contain plenty of omega-3 fatty acids, this dish is great as a healthy dessert or evening snack.

1. Place the millet in a small, dry saucepan over medium-high heat and toast for 2 to 3 minutes, until the color deepens slightly and it starts to smell toasty.

2. Transfer to a food processor (or blender). Add the chia seeds and ¼ cup of the slivered almonds, and pulse several times until the millet cracks and has the texture of whole grain flour.

3. Return the millet-almond mixture to the saucepan, along with the water, almond milk, vanilla, and salt. Reduce the heat to medium and simmer for 15 to 20 minutes, stirring frequently, until the millet softens and becomes creamy. Stir in the remaining ¼ cup slivered almonds.

4. Meanwhile, in a small saucepan, combine the blueberries and stevia. Cook, stirring slowly, until the blueberries defrost, 1 to 2 minutes.

5. Serve the millet porridge topped with the blueberries and additional almond milk (if using).

PER SERVING: CALORIES: 249; CARBS: 35G; GLYCEMIC LOAD: 16; FIBER: 6G; SODIUM: 76MG; PROTEIN: 7G; FAT: 10G; SATURATED FAT: 1G

Cherry Chia Pudding

INFLAMMATION FIGHTER, DAIRY FREE, GLUTEN FREE

2½ cups unsweetened almond milk

1 cup frozen unsweetened pitted dark cherries, thawed

½ teaspoon ground cardamom

½ teaspoon ground cinnamon

1 teaspoon vanilla extract

1 teaspoon powdered stevia

½ cup chia seeds

1 to 2 tablespoons sliced almonds, for garnish (optional)

SERVES 4 | PREP TIME: 25 MINUTES, PLUS 3 HOURS TO CHILL

Chia seeds are one of the richest plant sources of omega-3 fatty acids, a type of essential fat that can lower triglycerides and reduce your risk for heart disease. These tiny seeds are also full of slow-digesting, blood sugar–stabilizing fiber, bone-strengthening calcium and magnesium, and protein. Blended with phytonutrient-rich cherries, this creamy dessert will provide a boost of energy, help regulate your blood sugar, and keep you feeling full.

1. In a blender, combine the milk, cherries, cardamom, cinnamon, vanilla, and stevia and blend on high until smooth.

2. Place the chia seeds in a medium bowl, pour the cherry mixture over top, and whisk thoroughly to combine. Let the mixture rest for 5 minutes, then stir again. After 10 minutes, stir again. Cover and refrigerate for at least 3 hours or overnight.

3. Before serving, give the pudding another stir, then portion it evenly among 4 cups. Top with the sliced almonds (if using).

INFLAMMATION FIGHTER TIP: *This recipe uses cherries, a stone fruit rich in phytonutrients that have been shown through research to reduce inflammation, support healthy sleep, reduce belly fat, reduce post-exercise muscle pain, and lower the risk of stroke. Another equally nutritious fruit with its own unique set of plant nutrients is the blueberry. Consider mixing the two types of fruit to benefit from their synergy.*

PER SERVING: CALORIES: 217; CARBS: 24G; GLYCEMIC LOAD: 3; FIBER: 10G; SODIUM: 181MG; PROTEIN: 6G; FAT: 12G; SATURATED FAT: 1G

Cinnamon Bun Mug Cake

LOWER CALORIE, INFLAMMATION FIGHTER

1 egg

¼ cup old-fashioned
rolled oats

1 tablespoon coconut flour

1 tablespoon flaxseed meal

¼ teaspoon baking powder

¼ teaspoon ground nutmeg

¼ teaspoon vanilla extract

¼ teaspoon powdered stevia

1½ teaspoons ground
cinnamon, divided

Olive oil cooking spray

2 tablespoons nonfat vanilla
Greek yogurt

SERVES 1 | PREP TIME: 5 MINUTES | COOK TIME: 2 MINUTES

The texture of this healthy cinnamon bun treat is light and fluffy like a cake, but with a slight chewiness, making it a truly satisfying sweet snack, dessert, or even breakfast. And thanks to the protein from the egg, it won't cause a spike in blood sugar. Oil-free and delicious, this mug cake will soon be a go-to favorite.

1. Whisk the egg in a medium bowl. Add the oats, coconut flour, flaxseed meal, baking powder, nutmeg, vanilla, and stevia, and 1 teaspoon of the cinnamon; stir until well combined.

2. Coat a large coffee mug or ramekin with olive oil cooking spray. Pour the batter into the mug.

3. Microwave for 1 minute and 20 seconds or until the cake has puffed up and is no longer wet on top.

4. Top with the yogurt and sprinkle the remaining ½ teaspoon of cinnamon. The mug may be hot from the microwave, so take care.

INGREDIENT TIP: *For a more indulgent version, make an icing by stirring together 1 tablespoon coconut butter, 1 tablespoon water, and ¼ teaspoon stevia extract. Coconut butter is similar to coconut oil, but it contains some of the coconut meat itself. Note that this addition will add about 75 calories, mainly coming from fat.*

PER SERVING: CALORIES: 438; CARBS: 37G; GLYCEMIC LOAD: 17;
FIBER: 10G; SODIUM: 101MG; PROTEIN: 17G; FAT: 26G; SATURATED FAT: 16G

Peanut Butter Blondies

DAIRY FREE, GLUTEN FREE

Olive oil cooking spray
1 (15-ounce) can chickpeas
  (garbanzo beans), drained
  and rinsed
½ cup natural peanut butter
¼ cup brown rice syrup, or
  honey or agave syrup
¼ cup coconut sugar
2 tablespoons unsweetened
  almond milk
2 teaspoons vanilla extract
Pinch ground cinnamon
½ teaspoon salt
½ teaspoon baking powder
½ teaspoon baking soda

SERVES 9 | PREP TIME: 5 MINUTES, PLUS 15 MINUTES
COOLING TIME | COOK TIME 20 MINUTES

These healthy blondies taste indulgent, yet they are free of refined sugars and carbs, are vegan-friendly, and are actually good for you! The secret is replacing flour with chickpeas to produce a sweet treat that keeps your blood sugar steady by providing slow-digesting carbohydrates, ample protein, and a healthy dose of fiber. Perfectly moist and delicious, this dessert can be prepared in 30 minutes.

1. Preheat the oven to 350°F.

2. Coat a 9-inch square glass baking pan with olive oil cooking spray and set it aside.

3. In a food processor (or blender), combine the chickpeas, peanut butter, rice syrup, coconut sugar, almond milk, vanilla, cinnamon, salt, baking powder, and soda. Blend until creamy and smooth.

4. Pour the batter into the prepared pan and spread it out evenly.

5. Bake for 20 to 30 minutes, until the edges just pull away from the pan, the top is set, and the top is slightly golden brown.

6. Remove the pan from the oven and let the blondies cool for at least 15 minutes before slicing. Serve warm.

INGREDIENT TIP: *If you have a nut-free or peanut-free household, simply replace the peanut butter with non-GMO soy nut butter, sunflower seed butter, pumpkin butter, or another butter based on your preferences.*

PER SERVING: CALORIES: 195; CARBS: 25G; GLYCEMIC LOAD: 10; FIBER: 4G; SODIUM: 96MG; PROTEIN: 8G; FAT: 8G; SATURATED FAT: 2G

Chocolate Chip Cookie Dough Bites

DAIRY FREE, GLUTEN FREE

12 Medjool dates, pitted
½ cup chopped walnuts
1 tablespoon flaxseed meal
1 tablespoon hemp seeds
Pinch salt
¼ teaspoon ground cinnamon
1½ teaspoons vanilla extract
2 tablespoons mini
  chocolate chips

SERVES 18 BITES | PREP TIME: 10 MINUTES

There is a way to enjoy sweets while not having them wreak havoc on your body and cause surges in blood sugar. The trick is to be sure that they have a good balance of protein, fiber-rich carbohydrates, and fats, which will digest slowly and keep your blood sugar from rising and falling too quickly. These delicious cookie dough bites are high in anti-inflammatory omega-3 fats, fiber, and protein and made naturally sweet with Medjool dates.

1. In a food processor (or blender), combine the dates, walnuts, flaxseed meal, hemp seeds, salt, cinnamon, and vanilla; pulse until everything is well incorporated.

2. Spoon the batter into a medium bowl and fold in the chocolate chips. Roll the batter into 18 bite-size balls.

3. Store the cookie bites in an airtight container in the refrigerator for up to 4 days.

INFLAMMATION FIGHTER TIP: *This recipe lends well to variations, and you could easily increase its fiber, protein, vitamin, mineral, and omega-3 fatty acid content by adding 1 tablespoon of chia seeds.*

PER SERVING: CALORIES: 80; CARBS: 14G; GLYCEMIC LOAD: 7; FIBER: 2G; SODIUM: 0MG; PROTEIN: 1G; FAT: 3G; SATURATED FAT: 0G

Fudgy Black Bean Brownies

FERTILITY BOOST, INFLAMMATION FIGHTER, DAIRY FREE, GLUTEN FREE

Olive oil cooking spray

1 (15-ounce) can black beans, drained and rinsed

2 eggs

1 large cooked red beet, peeled and roughly chopped

½ cup raspberries

¼ cup coconut flour

1 tablespoon coconut oil, melted

¾ cup unsweetened cocoa powder

¼ teaspoon salt

1 teaspoon vanilla extract

1½ teaspoons baking powder

SERVES 9 | PREP TIME: 5 MINUTES | COOK TIME: 25 MINUTES

These healthy, fudgy black bean brownies have a secret ingredient that gives them an added touch of moisture and kicks the nutrition up a notch: a cooked red beet. Beets are loaded with vitamins A, B, and C and are high in fiber, manganese, folate, and phytonutrients called betalains, which have antioxidant and anti-inflammatory properties. High in fiber, protein, and health-promoting cocoa flavonols, these brownies will give you steady energy.

1. Preheat the oven to 350°F.

2. Lightly coat a 9-inch square baking pan with olive oil cooking spray.

3. In a food processor (or blender) bowl, combine the beans, eggs, beet, raspberries, coconut flour, coconut oil, cocoa powder, salt, vanilla, and baking powder. Purée for about 3 minutes, scraping down the sides of the bowl as needed, until smooth.

4. Spread the mixture into the prepared pan. Bake for 20 to 25 minutes or until the top is dry and the edges start to pull away from the sides.

5. Let cool on a rack for 30 minutes before slicing. The brownies will be tender, so remove them gently from the pan. The insides are intended to be moist and fudgy.

INGREDIENT TIP: *This recipe is sweetened using only raspberries, so if you want the brownies to be sweeter, try adding a little powdered stevia. You could also add coconut sugar, but note that this will raise the calorie count.*

PER SERVING: CALORIES: 154; CARBS: 21G; GLYCEMIC LOAD: 7; FIBER: 8G; SODIUM: 159MG; PROTEIN: 8G; FAT: 5G; SATURATED FAT: 3G

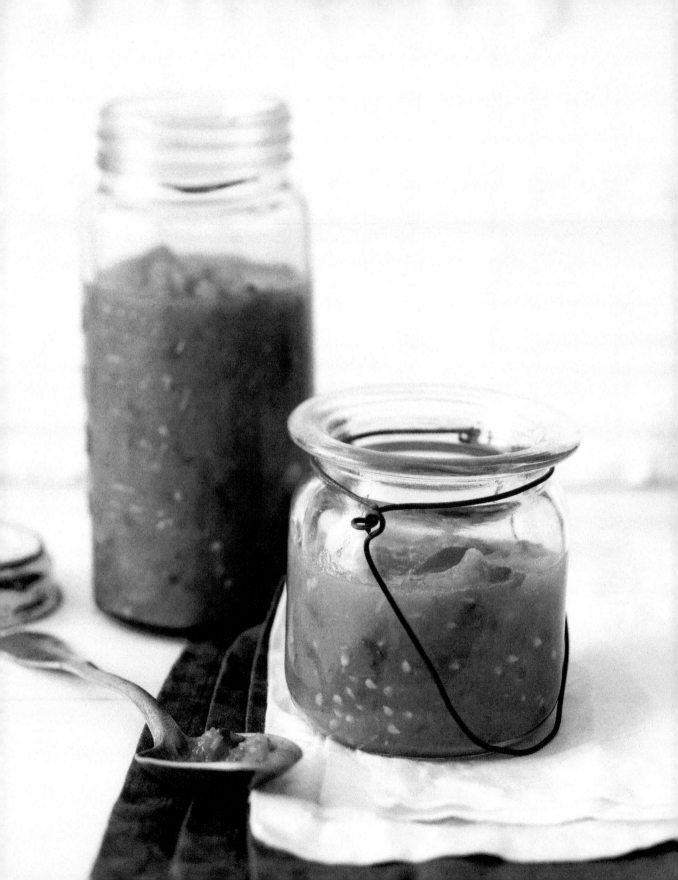

10

Broths, Sauces, and Dressings

Homemade Vegetable Broth

LOWER CALORIE, DAIRY FREE, GLUTEN FREE

4 medium carrots, peeled
  and roughly diced
4 celery stalks, roughly diced
2 large onions, roughly diced
4 medium garlic cloves,
  smashed
2 sprigs fresh flat-leaf parsley
2 sprigs fresh thyme
3 bay leaves
2 teaspoons whole black
  peppercorns
Salt

MAKES 8 CUPS | PREP TIME: 10 MINUTES | COOK TIME: 1 HOUR

This basic broth recipe is quick and easy, and far healthier than store-bought vegetable broth. Relying on simple ingredients, the recipe can be customized according to whatever vegetables you have on hand. This flavorful broth will enhance your favorite vegetarian soups or stews. To make stock instead of broth, simply omit the salt.

1. Place all the ingredients and 1 gallon water in a large soup pot over high heat. Bring to a boil. Reduce the heat to medium-low and simmer for 45 minutes to 1 hour.

2. Pour the broth through a fine mesh strainer into a large heatproof bowl or pot; discard the solids. Cool.

3. Transfer to airtight containers and refrigerate up to 3 days or in the freezer for up to 3 months. Stir before using if the broth separates.

INGREDIENT TIP: *In this flexible recipe, you don't need to use the specific vegetables listed in the amounts called for. Carrots, onions, and garlic should be used along with some type of herb. Celery is always good to add, as are leeks and fennel, if you have them.*

PER SERVING (1 CUP): CALORIES: 12; CARBS: 3G; GLYCEMIC LOAD: 0; FIBER: 0G; SODIUM: 32MG; PROTEIN: 0G; FAT: 0G; SATURATED FAT: 0G

Dairy-Free Pesto

INFLAMMATION FIGHTER, DAIRY FREE, GLUTEN FREE

3 cups gently packed
   fresh basil
½ cup blanched slivered
   almonds
Juice of 1 small lemon
2 large garlic cloves,
   roughly chopped
½ teaspoon salt
¼ cup extra-virgin olive oil,
   plus more if needed

MAKES 1 CUP | PREP TIME: 5 MINUTES

You may think the key to great pesto is aged Parmesan, but it is possible to create pesto perfection without dairy. Pesto making is one of those flexible, intuitive things that isn't an exact science. Just choose an herb or two (cilantro, basil, mint), a nut or seed (walnuts, hazelnuts, pine nuts, almonds), and a good-tasting oil. Pesto adds a flavor boost, healthy fats, and beneficial phytochemicals to all types of recipes, from grilled vegetables to egg dishes to pizza.

1. In a food processor (or blender), combine the basil, almonds, lemon juice, garlic, and salt; process into a coarse meal.

2. Slowly add the olive oil in a steady drizzle as you pulse the processor on and off. Process until a smooth, light paste forms. Add enough oil to keep the pesto moist and spreadable.

3. Store the pesto in an airtight container in the refrigerator for up to 5 days.

INGREDIENT TIP: *Lightly toasting the nuts before using them intensifies their flavor in just minutes. Think of the difference between granulated and caramelized sugar. You can toast the nuts on a baking sheet in a 350°F oven for 5 to 10 minutes, or in a dry pot on the stove top while stirring constantly for 5 to 10 minutes.*

PER SERVING (2 TABLESPOONS): CALORIES: 117; CARBS: 3G; GLYCEMIC LOAD: 0; FIBER: 1G; SODIUM: 149MG; PROTEIN: 2G; FAT: 11G; SATURATED FAT: 1G

Mushroom Gravy

LOWER CALORIE, INFLAMMATION FIGHTER, DAIRY FREE, GLUTEN FREE

1 cup low-sodium
   vegetable broth
2 tablespoons Bragg's
   liquid aminos
1 shallot, chopped
8 ounces mushrooms,
   stemmed and sliced
2 tablespoons
   arrowroot powder
2 tablespoons
   nutritional yeast
2 tablespoons minced
   fresh thyme
1 tablespoon minced fresh
   rosemary leaves
¼ teaspoon freshly ground
   black pepper

INFLAMMATION
FIGHTER TIP: *Shallots are a
type of onion, but they differ
in that they are smaller, they
grow in clusters of bulbs, and
the bulbs are less pungent than
onions and garlic. However, on
a per-weight basis, they have
more antioxidants, minerals,
and vitamins than onions do.
Consider increasing their quantity in this recipe to boost the
inflammation-fighting power.*

MAKES 2 CUPS | PREP TIME: 10 MINUTES | COOK TIME: 15 MINUTES

*This simple vegan gravy is easy to prepare using a variety of
different types of mushrooms and some basic pantry staples.
Store-bought gravy is usually high in sodium, unhealthy
fats, and preservatives; by preparing your own, you can
avoid unwanted ingredients and add valuable nutrients
to your diet. Mushrooms are high in vitamin D, a nutrient
many people are lacking, and they are also a rich source of
disease-protective antioxidants and phytochemicals. Try a
variety by combining cremini, button, shiitake, and more.
Enjoy this over tofu, veggie burgers, cooked grains, beans,
or vegetables, or stir some into greens for a hearty ragout.*

1. In a small saucepan over medium-high heat, combine
the broth and aminos and bring to a simmer. Turn the
heat to medium-low. Add the shallot and mushrooms,
and simmer gently for 10 minutes, stirring occasionally.

2. In a small bowl, stir the arrowroot powder with just
enough water to dissolve.

3. When the broth reaches a steady simmer, slowly
whisk in the arrowroot slurry, and stir constantly, until
the liquid thickens.

4. Remove the pan from the heat and whisk in the
nutritional yeast, thyme, rosemary, and pepper. Serve
immediately.

5. Store leftovers in an airtight jar in the refrigerator for
up to 3 days.

PER SERVING (¼ CUP): CALORIES: 23; CARBS: 4G; GLYCEMIC LOAD: 2;
FIBER: 1G; SODIUM: 322MG; PROTEIN: 2G; FAT: 0G; SATURATED FAT: 0G

Simple Tomato Sauce

LOWER CALORIE, INFLAMMATION FIGHTER, DAIRY FREE, GLUTEN FREE

2 tablespoons olive oil

1 medium onion,
    finely chopped

4 garlic cloves, minced

1 cup finely chopped celery

1 red bell pepper,
    finely chopped

10 ounces mushrooms,
    finely chopped

2 (28-ounce) cans crushed
    tomatoes with their juice

1 tablespoon chopped
    fresh basil

½ teaspoon dried oregano

Salt

Freshly ground black pepper

MAKES ABOUT 2 QUARTS | PREP TIME: 15 MINUTES
COOK TIME: 40 MINUTES

Most people don't have 2 hours to peel and cook fresh tomatoes and prepare an authentic red sauce from scratch. And while grocery stores have dozen of options available, you might be surprised to know that just about all of them contain high fructose corn syrup along with other less than healthy ingredients. You can make your own super-healthy sauce in about half an hour by using canned tomatoes and bumping up the nutrition with several different vegetables. High in vitamin C and phytochemicals, this delicious sauce is great over vegetable noodles, cooked grains, and beans.

1. Heat the olive oil in a large saucepan over medium-high heat. Add the onion, garlic, celery, bell pepper, and mushrooms and sauté until the onion is softened, 3 to 4 minutes.

2. Add the tomatoes, basil, and oregano, and season with salt and pepper. Bring the mixture to a simmer, reduce the heat to low, and simmer, stirring occasionally, for 30 to 40 minutes.

3. Serve hot.

4. Store the sauce in airtight containers in the refrigerator for up to 4 days, or in the freezer for up to 3 months.

COOKING TIP: *For a thinner sauce that works better for meats and poultry or pizza, purée the sauce using an immersion blender or blend it in a food processor (or blender) until smooth. Feel free to vary the vegetable ingredients based on what you have on hand. Other good options include butternut squash, spinach, and carrots.*

PER SERVING (½ CUP): CALORIES: 42; CARBS: 6G; GLYCEMIC LOAD: 2; FIBER: 1G; SODIUM: 17MG; PROTEIN: 2G; FAT: 2G; SATURATED FAT: 0G

Vegan Alfredo Sauce

DAIRY FREE, GLUTEN FREE

1 (13.5-ounce) can light
    coconut milk
½ cup nutritional yeast
¼ cup gently packed
    chopped fresh basil
2 garlic cloves, minced
1 teaspoon arrowroot powder
Salt
Freshly ground black pepper

MAKES ABOUT 2 CUPS | PREP TIME: 5 MINUTES
COOK TIME: 5 MINUTES

Traditional Alfredo sauce may taste good, but it isn't exactly good for the waistline or the heart. Made from butter, heavy cream, and Parmesan cheese, even a small portion is high in unhealthy fats and calories. If you have been looking for a healthy alternative, look no further than this dairy-free recipe, which is made with creamy coconut milk and cheesy-tasting, vitamin B–rich nutritional yeast.

1. In a food processor (or blender), combine the coconut milk, nutritional yeast, basil, and garlic; blend until smooth.

2. Pour into a medium saucepan over medium-high heat. Add the arrowroot and stir constantly until thickened. Season with salt and pepper.

3. Serve hot over vegetable noodles, cooked grains, beans, fish, poultry, or vegetables.

INGREDIENT TIP: *There are several ingredient variations you could use, based on your personal preferences: Replace the canned coconut milk with either 1 cup puréed cooked cauliflower and 1 cup almond milk, or 1 cup puréed silken tofu and 1 cup almond milk. Experiment and see which you prefer.*

PER SERVING (½ CUP): CALORIES: 212; CARBS: 11G; GLYCEMIC LOAD: 5; FIBER: 4G; SODIUM: 40MG; PROTEIN: 10G; FAT: 17G; SATURATED FAT: 15G

Blueberry Chia Sauce

INFLAMMATION FIGHTER, DAIRY FREE, GLUTEN FREE

2 cups fresh or frozen
  blueberries
½ to 1 cup water
2 tablespoons brown rice
  syrup, honey, or stevia
2 tablespoons chia seeds
1 to 2 tablespoons freshly
  squeezed lemon juice
  (optional)

COOKING TIP: *You can also make this recipe without cooking it. Simply mash the fruit with a fork until it is pulpy and juicy, and then stir in the rest of the ingredients. Uncooked chia sauce will be a bit looser, but you can add more chia seeds to get a thicker consistency, if wanted.*

YIELD 3 ¼ CUPS | PREP TIME: 5 MINUTES
COOK TIME: 10 MINUTES

Chia seeds bring the magic to this antioxidant- and phytochemical-rich berry sauce. Using the gelling powder of these tiny seeds, you can transform a few cups of fresh fruit into a low-sugar, spoonable sauce in about 15 minutes. Packed with omega-3 fats, fiber, and vitamins and minerals, this sauce is wonderful over waffles, swirled into smoothies, or poured over pudding. If you don't have blueberries, you can substitute raspberries, blackberries, or cranberries.

1. In a medium saucepan over medium-high heat, combine the berries, ½ cup of the water, and rice syrup, and heat, stirring frequently. When the mixture starts to simmer, reduce the heat to medium-low and let simmer for 5 minutes, while breaking down the berries with a wooden spoon. Leave some intact for texture.

2. Add the chia seeds and let the sauce thicken, stirring constantly, for 2 to 3 minutes. Add a bit more water, if needed, until the desired consistency is reached.

3. Remove the pan from the heat and let the sauce thicken for an additional 2 to 3 minutes.

4. Serve over waffles, pancakes, muffins, or Greek yogurt. Store in an airtight container in the refrigerator for up to 5 days.

PER SERVING (¼ CUP): CALORIES: 33; CARBS: 7G; GLYCEMIC LOAD: 3; FIBER: 1G; SODIUM: 1MG; PROTEIN: 1G; FAT: 1G; SATURATED FAT: 0G

Vegan Queso Sauce

FERTILITY BOOST, LOWER CALORIE, DAIRY FREE, GLUTEN FREE

1 cup unsweetened almond milk, plus more for thickness if needed

1 tablespoon gluten-free flour, plus more for thickness if needed

1 tablespoon olive oil

8 tablespoons nutritional yeast

2 teaspoons Dijon mustard

1 teaspoon Bragg's liquid aminos

½ teaspoon freshly ground black pepper

¼ teaspoon garlic powder

¼ teaspoon onion powder

Salt

FERTILITY BOOST TIP:

Consider making nutritional yeast a regular part of your cooking for additional fertility-boosting nutrients. A 2-tablespoon serving of nutritional yeast provides 60 percent of the recommended daily value for folate, and 6 times the daily value for a number of other B vitamins. You will find this ingredient at health food stores, online retailers, and in the baking aisle or bulk bins section at supercenter and grocery stores.

MAKES ¾ CUP | PREP TIME: 5 MINUTES | COOK TIME: 10 MINUTES

When that craving for cheese strikes, whip up this creamy vegan queso in minutes with a few basic ingredients. Dairy cheese is an excellent source of protein, calcium, and vitamin D, but with those nutrients comes the price of added salt and unhealthy types of fats. Vegan cheese has no harmful fats and truly has a taste and texture so similar to dairy cheese you won't believe it. This sauce is high in B vitamins and protein, with added calcium from the almond milk, and is especially delicious in lasagna, mac and cheese, or drizzled over steamed veggies.

1. In a medium bowl, whisk together the milk and gluten-free flour until smooth.

2. Heat the olive oil in a medium skillet over medium heat. Add the milk mixture and the nutritional yeast and whisk well. Reduce the heat to medium-low.

3. Add the mustard, aminos, pepper, garlic powder, and onion powder, season with salt, and cook, whisking frequently, until the sauce thickens, about 5 minutes. Add more milk or flour to achieve the thickness you desire, if needed.

4. Store in an airtight container for 5 to 7 days. Reheat in the microwave or on the stove top before using.

PER SERVING (¼ CUP): CALORIES: 132; CARBS: 12G; GLYCEMIC LOAD: 3; FIBER: 6G; SODIUM: 235MG; PROTEIN: 11G; FAT: 6G; SATURATED FAT: 1G

Sesame Ginger Miso Dressing

LOWER CALORIE, INFLAMMATION FIGHTER, DAIRY FREE

½ to ¾ cup water

½ cup miso

2 tablespoons rice vinegar

2 tablespoons low-sodium soy sauce

2 tablespoons sesame oil

3 garlic cloves, minced

1 teaspoon peeled and minced fresh ginger

½ teaspoon onion powder

MAKES 1½ CUPS | PREP TIME: 5 MINUTES

Miso is a paste made from soybeans, sea salt, and koji (a mold starter) that is allowed to ferment for 3 months to 3 years, producing an enzyme-rich food loaded with beneficial microorganisms. High in antioxidants that protect against free radical damage, B vitamins, and isoflavones (phytoestrogens), miso adds a deep flavor to a variety of dishes. Here it is used to create a simple and nutritious dressing that adds a flavorful punch to salads, steamed veggies, and cooked poultry and tofu. To control the consistency of this dressing, add more or less water.

1. In a blender, combine the water, miso, vinegar, soy sauce, sesame oil, garlic, ginger, and onion powder. Blend until smooth.

2. Store the dressing in the refrigerator in an airtight container up to 4 days.

INFLAMMATION FIGHTER TIP: *Most dressings require a thickening ingredient, and here, sesame oil is used for that purpose. Other healthy thickeners that would work well in this recipe and add more nutrients include: tahini, avocado, tofu, shelled sunflower seeds, cooked beans, carrots, or winter squash.*

PER SERVING (2 TABLESPOONS): CALORIES: 46; CARBS: 3G; GLYCEMIC LOAD: 2; FIBER: 1G; SODIUM: 595MG; PROTEIN: 2G; FAT: 3G; SATURATED FAT: 0G

Hemp Seed Dressing

INFLAMMATION FIGHTER, DAIRY FREE, GLUTEN FREE

¾ cup hemp seeds

¾ cup water, plus more
  if needed

2 pitted dates

3 garlic cloves, minced

1 tablespoon apple
  cider vinegar

2 tablespoons freshly
  squeezed lemon juice

1 teaspoon dill

Salt

Freshly ground black pepper

INFLAMMATION
FIGHTER TIP: *Hemp seeds,
also known as hemp hearts,
are one of the most nutritious
seeds you can eat. They are
incredibly small, which makes
incorporating them into your
diet easy because you can
add them to so many things.
Use them in smoothies, chia
pudding, on top of cooked vegetables and grains, as a salad
or cereal topper, on top of oatmeal, in pancakes and baked
goods, and so much more!*

MAKES 2 CUPS | PREP TIME: 5 MINUTES, PLUS 2 TO 3 HOURS
OF SOAKING TIME

*It's so much easier and healthier to make your own salad
dressing at home. You can tailor the ingredients to your
palate and control the amounts of salt and sugar. This creamy
dressing doesn't contain any oil or dairy and instead gets its
thick consistency from hemp seeds. Hemp seeds are high in
protein, fiber, antioxidants, and important essential omega-3
fats, which decrease inflammation in the body. Serve this
dressing in wraps or over salads, veggies, and cooked grains
and beans.*

1. Put the hemp seeds in a medium bowl and cover
with water. Soak for 2 to 3 hours at room temperature
or overnight in the refrigerator.

2. Drain the seeds in a sieve and rinse until the water
runs clear.

3. In a blender, put the hemp seeds, the water, dates,
garlic, vinegar, and lemon juice and blend until smooth.
Pour into a medium bowl.

4. Whisk in the dill and season with salt and pepper.

5. Store the dressing in an airtight container in the
refrigerator for up to 4 days.

PER SERVING (2 TABLESPOONS): CALORIES: 40; CARBS: 6G;
GLYCEMIC LOAD: 1; FIBER: 0G; SODIUM: 6MG; PROTEIN: 2G; FAT: 2G;
SATURATED FAT: 0G

Strawberry Vinaigrette

FERTILITY BOOST, LOWER CALORIE, INFLAMMATION FIGHTER, DAIRY FREE, GLUTEN FREE

2 cups fresh strawberries

2 tablespoons
balsamic vinegar

1 tablespoon
red wine vinegar

1 tablespoon freshly
squeezed lemon juice

1 garlic clove, smashed

¼ teaspoon mustard powder

1 tablespoon olive oil

1 tablespoon honey
(optional)

Salt

Freshly ground black pepper

MAKES 1⅓ CUPS | PREP TIME: 5 MINUTES

Nutrient-rich and packed with vitamin C, folate, and several minerals, the juicy, delicious strawberry is the main ingredient in this healthy, low-calorie vinaigrette. The bright red color of strawberries comes from their anthocyanidin content, a phytonutrient thought to protect against inflammation, cancer, and heart disease. High in blood sugar–stabilizing fiber, this simple strawberry vinaigrette is a healthy alternative to store-bought dressings.

1. In a blender, combine the strawberries, balsamic vinegar, red wine vinegar, lemon juice, garlic, mustard, olive oil, and honey (if using), and season with salt and pepper. Blend until smooth.

2. Serve immediately or store in an airtight container in the refrigerator for up to 4 days.

INGREDIENT TIP: *If possible, choose organic strawberries to reduce exposure to pesticide residue. If they aren't in season, choose frozen organic unsweetened strawberries and allow them to thaw in the refrigerator before using.*

PER SERVING (2 TABLESPOONS): CALORIES: 27; CARBS: 3G; GLYCEMIC LOAD: 1; FIBER: 1G; SODIUM: 11MG; PROTEIN: 0G; FAT: 1G; SATURATED FAT: 0G

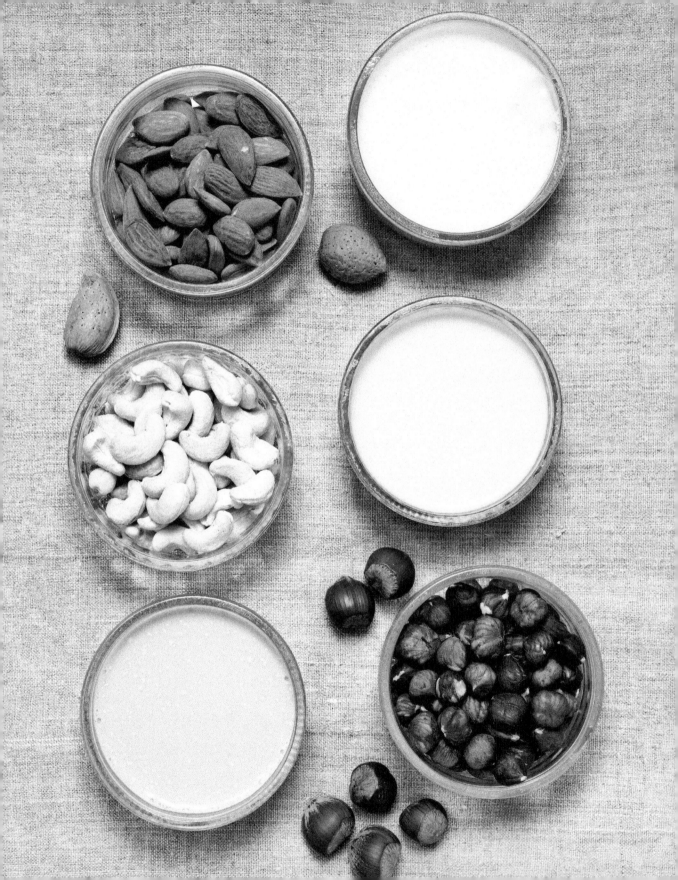

APPENDIX A: GLYCEMIC INDEX AND GLYCEMIC LOAD FOOD LIST

The following is a list of the glycemic index and glycemic load rankings of many common carbohydrates. Foods are ranked between 0 and 100 based on how they affect one's blood glucose level. The best choices are low or medium on the glycemic index, with a rating of 55 to 69.

Remember that it is more important to pay attention to the glycemic load of a food—that is, the amount of carbohydrates it contains per serving. The best choices have low (less than 10) or moderate (between 10 and 20) glycemic loads.

FOOD	GLYCEMIC INDEX	SERVING SIZE (GRAMS)	GLYCEMIC LOAD (PER SERVING)
BAKERY PRODUCTS			
Bagel, white	72	70	25
Baguette, white	95	30	15
Barley bread	34	30	7
Corn tortilla	52	50	12
Croissant	67	57	17
Doughnut	76	47	17
Pita bread	68	30	10
Sourdough rye	48	30	6
Soya & linseed bread	36	30	3
Sponge cake	46	63	17
Wheat tortilla	30	50	8
White wheat flour bread	71	30	10
Whole wheat bread	71	30	9

FOOD	GLYCEMIC INDEX	SERVING SIZE (GRAMS)	GLYCEMIC LOAD (PER SERVING)
BEVERAGES			
Apple juice, unsweetened	44	250 mL	30
Coca-Cola	63	250 mL	16
Gatorade	78	250 mL	12
Lucozade	95	250 mL	40
Orange juice, unsweetened	50	250 mL	12
Tomato juice, canned	38	250 mL	4
BREAKFAST CEREALS			
All-Bran	55	30	12
Cocoa Krispies	77	30	20
Cornflakes	93	30	23
Muesli, average	66	30	16
Oatmeal, average	55	50	13
Special K	69	30	14
DAIRY			
Ice cream, regular	57	50	6
Milk, full fat	41	250 mL	5
Milk, skim	32	250 mL	4
Reduced-fat yogurt with fruit	33	200	11
FRUITS			
Apple	39	120	6
Banana, ripe	62	120	16

FOOD	GLYCEMIC INDEX	SERVING SIZE (GRAMS)	GLYCEMIC LOAD (PER SERVING)
Cherries	22	120	3
Dates, dried	42	60	18
Grapefruit	25	120	3
Grapes	59	120	11
Mango	41	120	8
Orange	40	120	4
Peach	42	120	5
Pear	38	120	4
Pineapple	51	120	8
Raisins	64	60	28
Strawberries	40	120	1
Watermelon	72	120	4

GRAINS

FOOD	GLYCEMIC INDEX	SERVING SIZE (GRAMS)	GLYCEMIC LOAD (PER SERVING)
Brown rice	50	150	16
Buckwheat	45	150	13
Bulgur	30	50	11
Corn on the cob	60	150	20
Couscous	65	150	9
Fettuccini, average	32	180	15
Gnocchi	68	180	33
Macaroni, average	47	180	23
Quinoa	53	150	13
Spaghetti, white	46	180	22

FOOD	GLYCEMIC INDEX	SERVING SIZE (GRAMS)	GLYCEMIC LOAD (PER SERVING)
Spaghetti, whole wheat	42	180	26
Vermicelli noodles	35	180	16
White rice	89	150	43

LEGUMES

FOOD	GLYCEMIC INDEX	SERVING SIZE (GRAMS)	GLYCEMIC LOAD (PER SERVING)
Baked beans	40	150	6
Black beans	30	150	7
Butter beans	36	150	8
Chickpeas	10	150	3
Kidney beans	29	150	7
Lentils	29	150	5
Navy beans	31	150	9
Soy beans	50	150	1

SNACK FOODS

FOOD	GLYCEMIC INDEX	SERVING SIZE (GRAMS)	GLYCEMIC LOAD (PER SERVING)
Cashews, salted	27	50	3
Corn chips, plain, salted	42	50	11
Fruit Roll-Ups	99	30	24
Graham crackers	74	25	14
Honey	61	25	12
Hummus	6	30	0
M&M's, peanut	33	30	6
Microwave popcorn, plain	55	20	6
Muesli bar	61	30	13
Nutella	33	20	4

FOOD	GLYCEMIC INDEX	SERVING SIZE (GRAMS)	GLYCEMIC LOAD (PER SERVING)
Peanuts	7	50	0
Potato chips, average	51	50	12
Pretzels	83	30	16
Rice cakes	82	25	17
Rye crisps	64	25	11
Shortbread	64	25	10
Vanilla wafers	77	25	14
Walnuts	15	28	0
VEGETABLES			
Beets	64	80	4
Carrot	35	80	2
Green peas	51	80	4
Parsnip	52	80	4
Sweet potato, average	70	150	22
White potato, boiled	81	150	22
Yam	54	150	20

Sources: Harvard Health Publications (www.health.harvard.edu/healthy-eating/glycemic_index_and _glycemic_load_for_100_foods) and Mendosa.com (www.mendosa.com/gilists.htm).

APPENDIX B: CONVERSION TABLES

Volume Equivalents (Liquid)

US STANDARD	US STANDARD (OUNCES)	METRIC (APPROXIMATE)
2 tablespoons	1 fl. oz.	30 mL
¼ cup	2 fl. oz.	60 mL
½ cup	4 fl. oz.	120 mL
1 cup	8 fl. oz.	240 mL
1½ cups	12 fl. oz.	355 mL
2 cups or 1 pint	16 fl. oz.	475 mL
4 cups or 1 quart	32 fl. oz.	1 L
1 gallon	128 fl. oz.	4 L

Oven Temperatures

FAHRENHEIT (F)	CELSIUS (C) (APPROXIMATE)
250°F	120°C
300°F	150°C
325°F	165°C
350°F	180°C
375°F	190°C
400°F	200°C
425°F	220°C
450°F	230°C

Volume Equivalents (Dry)

US STANDARD	METRIC (APPROXIMATE)
¼ teaspoon	1 mL
½ teaspoon	2 mL
1 teaspoon	5 mL
1 tablespoon	15 mL
¼ cup	59 mL
⅓ cup	79 mL
½ cup	118 mL
1 cup	235 mL

Weight Equivalents

US STANDARD	METRIC (APPROXIMATE)
½ ounce	15 g
1 ounce	30 g
2 ounces	60 g
4 ounces	115 g
8 ounces	225 g
12 ounces	340 g
16 ounces or 1 pound	455 g

APPENDIX C: THE DIRTY DOZEN AND THE CLEAN FIFTEEN

A nonprofit and environmental watchdog organization called the Environmental Working Group (EWG) looks at data supplied by the US Department of Agriculture (USDA) and the Food and Drug Administration (FDA) about pesticide residues. Each year it compiles a list of the lowest and highest pesticide loads found in commercial crops. You can use these lists to decide which fruits and vegetables to buy organic to minimize your exposure to pesticides and which produce is considered safe enough to buy conventionally. This does not mean they are pesticide-free, though, so wash these fruits and vegetables thoroughly.

These lists change every year, so make sure you look up the most recent one before you fill your shopping cart. You'll find the most recent lists as well as a guide to pesticides in produce at EWG.org/FoodNews.

THE DIRTY DOZEN

- Apples
- Celery
- Cherry tomatoes
- Cucumbers
- Grapes
- Nectarines (imported)
- Peaches
- Potatoes
- Snap peas (imported)
- Spinach
- Strawberries
- Sweet bell peppers

Kale/Collard greens & Hot peppers*

THE CLEAN FIFTEEN

- Asparagus
- Avocados
- Cabbage
- Cantaloupes (domestic)
- Cauliflower
- Eggplants
- Grapefruits
- Kiwis
- Mangoes
- Onions
- Papayas
- Pineapples
- Sweet corn
- Sweet peas (frozen)
- Sweet potatoes

*In addition to the Dirty Dozen, the EWG added two produce items contaminated with highly toxic organo-phosphate insecticides.

ACKNOWLEDGMENTS

From Tara

I would like to thank my closest friends for being so supportive during the time of my own PCOS diagnosis, which allowed me to find the strength to tackle this condition. My friends taught me to stop expecting perfection in myself, and helped me nourish my body from the inside out. I am also grateful to the new friendships I have built with other PCOS sufferers, and I hope that my work has helped them as much as their wonderful support has helped me.

I'm thankful to my terrific editor, Clara Song Lee, for always being a pleasure to work with, along with the entire team at Callisto Media. And thank you to my coauthor, Jennifer Koslo, for producing so many delicious recipes, which I have added to my meal rotation.

From Jennifer

My sincere thanks and appreciation to my clients for teaching me about their struggles with insulin resistance and PCOS. Working with them has made me a more effective registered dietitian and nutritionist.

I also want to thank the thousands of registered dietitian and nutrition professionals working on the front lines every day, in clinics, hospitals, offices, and research laboratories, helping make a difference in the way people eat and live their lives. Every day, my colleagues inspire me to advance the field.

I am also deeply grateful to my editor, Clara Song Lee, for choosing such a meaningful topic for publication.

And I want to thank my family for their continued love, support, and encouragement.

RESOURCES

The resources listed below are excellent sites for obtaining more information on PCOS, insulin resistance, self-compassion, and positive body image.

The American Psychological Associaton (APA) provides a list of qualified therapists in your area, categorized by expertise and credentials. www.apa.org/helpcenter /choose-therapist.aspx.

Beauty Redefined is a website that aims to challenge beauty norms in the media, and positively change people's perceptions of their bodies. www.beautyredefined.net.

The Center for Young Women's Health is for younger women who struggle with poor self-esteem and body image. The website incudes resources for PCOS sufferers. www.youngwomenshealth.org/2012/05/30 /self-esteem.

The Insulin Resistance Diet Plan and Cookbook is a book Tara wrote in 2015, which provides further details about insulin resistance and how to manage it through diet and lifestyle changes. It is a great sister book for this book. www.amazon.com /Insulin-Resistance-Diet-Plan-Cookbook /dp/1623157285.

The **Intuitive Eating** website addresses intuitive eating and offers instructions for commencing an intuitive eating process and eating more mindfully. www.intuitiveeating.com.

Momentum and **Productive** are mobile applications that act as electronic habit trackers. They are available for iOS and Android phones.

The National Eating Disorders Association is a nonprofit organization for those who are affected by eating disorders. It features a great amount of information for building a healthy body image. www.nationaleatingdisorders.org /developing-and-maintaining -positive-body-image.

The National Institute of Diabetes and Digestive and Kidney Diseases website explains how insulin resistance and prediabetes develop, for those who would like to gain a better scientific understanding of their condition. www.niddk.nih.gov /health-information/health-topics/Diabetes /insulin-resistance-prediabetes.

The Natural Fertility Info website contains a comprehensive list of what dietary supplements can help improve PCOS, and why. www.natural-fertility-info.com /pcos-fertility-diet.

The PCOS Awareness Association is a nonprofit organization that aims to spread awareness about PCOS by increasing early diagnosis rates and overcoming the various individual symptoms of the condition. It links to a number of support groups worldwide. www.pcosaa.org.

The PCOS Diet Support group is a community of women who are affected by PCOS. Within this Facebook group, the women share articles, general tips, and positive mantras to help each other overcome their PCOS. www.facebook.com /PCOSDietSupport.

The PCOS Support Group is an active community with almost 20,000 members who suffer from PCOS. www.pcos .supportgroups.com.

Self-Compassion is a website operated by Kristen Neff, PhD, which includes written, spoken, and meditative exercises to help you practice self-compassion. www.self-compassion.org.

REFERENCES

American Heart Association. "Managing Blood Pressure with a Heart-Healthy Diet." Last modified October 23, 2015. Accessed November 26, 2015. www.heart.org/HEARTORG /Conditions/HighBloodPressure /PreventionTreatmentofHighBlood Pressure/Managing-Blood -Pressure-with-a-Heart-Healthy -Diet_UCM_301879 _Article.jsp#.WELhurn3E20.

Biaggioni, I., and S. Davis. "Caffeine: A Cause of Insulin Resistance?" *Diabetes Care* 25, no. 2 (February 2002): 399–400.

Chetty, S., Friedman, A., Taravosh-Lahn, K., Kirby, E., Mirescu, C., Guo, F., Krupik, D., et al. "Stress and Glucocorticoids Promote Oligodendrogenesis in the Adult Hippocampus." *Molecular Psychiatry* 19, no. 12 (December 2014): 1275–1283.

Cohen, D., Wang, W., Wyatt, J., Kronauer, R., Dijk, D., Czeisler, C., and Klerman, E. "Uncovering Residual Effects of Chronic Sleep Loss on Human Performance." *Science Translational Medicine* 2, no. 14 (January 2010): 14.

Colberg, S., Sigal, R., Fernhall, B., Regensteiner, J., Blissmer, B., Rubin, R., Chasan-Taber, L., Allbright, A., and B. Braun. "Exercise and Type 2 Diabetes." *Diabetes Care* 33, no. 12 (December 2010): 147–167.

Dunaif, A. "Insulin Resistance and the Polycystic Ovary Syndrome: Mechanism and Implications for Pathogenesis." *Endocrine Reviews* 18, no. 6 (1997): 774–800.

Grassi, A. "Soy and PCOS: Safe or Harmful?" PCOS Nutrition Center. Accessed November 17, 2016. www.pcosnutrition .com/2068/.

Healthy Line. "Testosterone Levels by Age." Accessed October 4, 2016. www.healthline.com/health/low -testosterone/testosterone-levels-by-age.

Healthy Women. "Polycystic Ovary Syndrome." Last modified December 2, 2015. Accessed October 2, 2016. www.healthywomen.org/condition /polycystic-ovary-syndrome.

Hutchinson, P. "How Many Calories a Day Does the Average Body Burn?" Livestrong. Last modified February 7, 2014. Accessed October 2, 2016. www.livestrong.com/article /315121-how-many-calories-a-day -does-the-average-body-burn.

Hutchinson, S., Stepto, N., Harrison, C., Moran, B., and Teede, H. "Effects of Exercise on Insulin Resistance and Body Composition in Overweight and Obese Women With and Without Polycystic Ovary Syndrome." *The Journal of Clinical Endocrinology and Metabolism* 96, no. 1 (April 2011): 48–56.

Kiddy, D., Hamilton-Fairley, D., Bush, A., Short, F., Anyaoku, V., Reed, M., and Franks, S. "Improvement in Endocrine and Ovarian Function During Dietary Treatment of Obese Women With Polycystic Ovary Syndrome." *Clinical Endocrinology (Oxford)* 36, no. 1 (January 1992): 105–111.

Kondracki, N. "The Link Between Sleep and Weight Gain—Research Shows Poor Sleep Quality Raises Obesity and Chronic Disease Risk." *Today's Dietitian* 14, no. 6 (June 2012): 48.

Lally, P., Jaarsveld, C., Potts, H., and Wardle, J. "How Are Habits Formed: Modelling Habit Formation in the Real World." *European Journal of Social Psychology* 40, no. 6 (October 2010): 998–1009.

Livingstone, C., and Collison, M. "Sex Steroids and Insulin Resistance." *Clinical Science* 102, no. 2 (February 2002): 151–156.

Mori, A. M., Considine, R.V., and Mattes, R. D., "Acute and Second Meal-Effects of Almond Form in Impaired Glucose Tolerant Adults: A Randomized Crossover Trial." *Nutrition & Metabolism*, 2011. Doi: 10.1186/1743-7075-8-6.

National Center for Complementary and Integrative Health (NCCIH). Garlic. Updated September 2016. Accessed November 4, 2016. https://nccih.nih.gov/health/garlic/ataglance.htm.

Natural Fertility Info. "How to Reduce the Damaging Effects of PCOS on Fertility Through Diet and Herbs." Accessed October 6, 2016. www.natural-fertility-info.com/pcos-fertility-diet.

Nestler, J., Jakubowicz, D., de Vargas, A., Brik, C., Quintero, N., and Medina, F. "Insulin Stimulates Testosterone Biosynthesis by Human Thecal Cells from Women with Polycystic Ovary Syndrome by Activating Its Own Receptor and Using Inositolglycan Mediators as the Signal Transduction System." *The Journal of Clinical Endocrinology and Metabolism* 83, no. 6 (June 1998): 2001–2005.

Putterman, E., and Linden, W. "Cognitive Dietary Restraint and Cortisol: Importance of Pervasive Concerns with Appearance." *Appetite* 47, no. 1 (July 2006): 64–76.

Roberts, S., and Dallal, G. "Energy Requirements and Aging." *Public Health Nutrition* 8, no. 7a (October 2005): 1028–1036.

Stepto, N., Cassar, S., Joham, A., Hutchinson, S., Harrison, C., Goldstein, R., and Teede, H. "Women with Polycystic Ovary Syndrome Have Intrinsic Insulin Resistance on Euglycaemic-Hyperinsulaemic Clamp." *Human Reproduction* 28, no. 3 (March 2013): 777–784.

Thomson, R. L., Spedding, S., and Buckley, J. D. "Vitamin D in the Aetiology and Management of Polycystic Ovary Syndrome." *Clinical Endocrinology*, 77, no. 3 (2012): 343–350.

US Department of Health and Human Services. 2015-2020 Dietary Guidelines for Americans. Accessed October 19, 2016. https://health.gov /dietaryguidelines/2015/

Wien, M., Haddad E., Oda K., Sabaté J. "A Randomized 3x3 Crossover Study to Evaluate the Effect of Hass Avocado Intake on Post-Ingestive Satiety, Glucose and Insulin Levels, and Subsequent Energy Intake in Overweight Adults." *Nutrition Journal,* 2013. Doi: 10.1186/1475-2891-12-155.

Women's Health. "Polycystic Ovary Syndrome." Last modified June 8, 2016. Accessed October 5, 2016. www.womenshealth.gov/publications /our-publications/fact-sheet /polycystic-ovary-syndrome.html#a.

RECIPE INDEX

INDEX

ABOUT THE AUTHORS

As a Fitness-Industry-Education-qualified nutritionist and certified personal trainer, **Tara Spencer** guides people on their path toward good health. She is experienced with eating disorder recovery, athlete coaching, and utilizing diet as a natural treatment for a number of illnesses. Her work as a nutritionist has given her the opportunity to impact a wide range of people of all ages and stages, from committed and recovering couch potatoes to novice bodybuilding competitors and professional tennis players. She is the author of two previous nutrition books: *The Insulin Resistance Diet Plan and Cookbook*, and *The Migraine Relief Diet*. To learn more about Tara, visit her online at www.sweatlikeapig.com.

Jennifer Koslo is a Registered Dietitian Nutritionist, Board Certified Specialist in Sports Dietetics, Licensed Dietitian in the state of Texas, and an American Council on Exercise Certified Personal Trainer. A member of the Sports, Cardiovascular, and Wellness Practice Group of the Academy of Nutrition and Dietetics (SCAN), she holds a PhD in education and a dual Master of Science degree in Exercise Science and Human Nutrition. Jennifer's experience includes almost three years as a US Peace Corps fisheries volunteer in Sierra Leone, West Africa; working as a cardiac dietitian for a state health department; teaching college-level nutrition and sports nutrition; providing individual nutrition counseling; and offering personal training services. She is the author of four previous healthy eating cookbooks: *The 21-Day Healthy Smoothie Plan*, *Diabetic Cooking for Two*, *The Healthy Smoothie Recipe Book*, and *The Alkaline Diet for Beginners*.

CPSIA information can be obtained
at www.ICGtesting.com
Printed in the USA
BVOW11s1228200117

473721BV00001B/1/P